GUY DEACON CBE jc [barcode] He
spent 18 months in the Democratic Republic of the Congo
with the UN disarming and demobilising rebel forces, for
which he was awarded an OBE; he was later awarded a CBE
for strategic work as Colonel of the Royal Armoured Corps.
Guy was diagnosed with Parkinson's in 2010, but carried on
working until the age of 57; he now has advanced Parkinson's.
As an ambassador for Cure Parkinson's and Parkinson's Africa,
Guy has visited twenty-five African countries to spotlight the
issues associated with Parkinson's disease in Africa. Guy lives
in Dorset with his wife and their dog, and continues in his
mission to raise awareness and provide support for people with
Parkinson's worldwide.

'An immense feat of endurance, a remarkable achievement, and a truly inspirational adventure filled with courage and hope.'

Sir Ranulph Fiennes

'Guy Deacon is a true hero. For over thirteen years, he has battled with Parkinson's disease. This is one of the cruellest illnesses in the world, which slowly saps one's strength and for which there is no cure – yet.

'Realising he could be nearing his end, Guy Deacon left his loving family and set out on an incredible journey to drive on his own, 18,000 miles across Europe and the full length of Africa.

'On his travels, Guy kept a video diary capturing the passing countryside and the locals who came to his aid. He was also helped, on several occasions, by a documentary maker.

'This has resulted in a Channel 4 documentary, which will create massive publicity for the horrors of Parkinson's disease and hopefully raise vast amounts of money and awareness to enable the medical profession to finally find a cure.

'I myself speak from bitter experience, because my darling husband, Leo Cooper, a great athlete and publisher of wonderful military history books, died from Parkinson's disease in 2013, two years after we celebrated our golden wedding anniversary. This meant that I and our children had the nightmare of watching him slowly disintegrate, despite him, like Guy Deacon, facing his failing abilities with huge courage.

'So please everyone, make sure you read *Running on Empty* by Guy Deacon.

'We must do everything we can in the world to raise the funds to find a cure.'

Jilly Cooper DBE

'Guy Deacon's inspirational journey through Africa is enthralling. With an indomitable spirit, Guy battles terrible roads, hostile border officials, mechanical breakdowns, but, most of all, Parkinson's disease – as he travels 18,000 miles, raising awareness and dispelling myths about a condition which is often stigmatised.'

Rory Cellan-Jones

RUNNING ON EMPTY

18,000 Miles Down Africa with Parkinson's

GUY DEACON

First published in the UK in 2024 by Ad Lib Publishers Ltd
Marine House, Tide Mill Way,
Woodbridge, Suffolk IP12 1AP

Text © 2024 Guy Deacon

Paperback ISBN 9781802471885
eBook ISBN 9781802472271

A CIP catalogue record for this book is
available from the British Library.

Every reasonable effort has been made to trace copyright-
holders of material reproduced in this book, but if any have
been inadvertently overlooked the publishers would be glad to
hear from them.

Printed in the UK
10 9 8 7 6 5 4 3 2 1

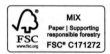

This book is dedicated to those special people in this world who have given up so much to care for loved ones struggling with Parkinson's disease. They too are victims; they too suffer. Worse still, they carry the burden of responsibility for the wellbeing of someone else. Despite their best efforts, they are helpless in stemming the tide of this debilitating disease and have to look on as their nearest and dearest relentlessly deteriorate. But it is the love, strength and support of these special people that makes Parkinson's 'long road' more bearable.

Contents

CONTENTS

1

The Diagnosis

The neurologist looked at me, his face impassive.

'I have good news and bad news. The good news is you have Parkinson's. There are pills to control it and it won't kill you.'

He paused, assuming I was going to ask what the bad news was.

I didn't. So he continued.

'The bad news is there's no cure and it's going to get worse.'

The entire examination at the James Cook hospital in Middlesbrough had taken less than ten minutes. The neurologist had done some simple tests, such as making me tie my shoelaces, walk three paces to the door and open and close my fingers and thumbs like they were ducks quacking. He gave his diagnosis matter of factly, which I suppose is the best way to do it when you are telling someone they will spend the rest of their lives in an incurably and increasingly debilitated state.

But even so, I clung to a last shred of hope. 'Are you sure?'

He nodded. 'I'll bet my reputation on it. Just take the pills and you'll be fine.'

He then gave me a prescription for Sinemet and Pramipexole dopamine enhancer pills, and that was me done. I walked out of the building and joined a group of people in the smoking shelter, and scrounged a light off one. All my fellow smokers were also suffering from some sort of medical problem. I had a moment of self-pity and briefly wept. 'Why me? I'm only forty-nine years old.'

Parkinson's disease is caused by a loss of nerve cells in a part of the brain called the substantia nigra. This leads to a reduction in a chemical called dopamine, which plays a vital role in regulating the movement of the body. A reduction in dopamine is responsible for many of the symptoms of Parkinson's disease, including involuntary tremors or shaking, slow movement, stiff and inflexible muscles, chronic lack of coordination and a host of psychological problems such as depression and anxiety. Exactly what causes the loss of nerve cells is unclear. What is clear is that at the moment there is no cure.

I had heard of Parkinson's, of course. I knew that Muhammad Ali and the American actor Michael J. Fox had it. But I never thought it would happen to me.

In the car going home, I phoned my wife, Tania. I told her I had Parkinson's, but was otherwise absolutely fine and it was no big deal. Nothing to worry about, I said. I deliberately made light of it, and that was the way I was going to handle the situation. I would carry on as normally as possible. And I wouldn't trouble anybody else with it. Despite seeming somewhat flippant, I was shocked to my core. But I suppose I should not have been that stunned as I had known – subliminally or not – that something odd had been going on with my coordination for some time. The first signs appeared when I was sent to the Democratic Republic of the Congo (DRC) as a colonel in the British Army in 2010 on what was to become an eighteen-month operational tour with the peacekeeping mission run by the United Nations (UN). The eastern part of that vast, chaotic country was still recovering from the Second Congo War, also known as the Great War of Africa, that claimed 5.4 million lives and displaced two million others. It was the deadliest conflict anywhere on the planet since the Second World War.

I had been appointed the UN Peacekeeping's Deputy Chief of Staff (Forward) and was based in the frontline conflict city of Goma on the Rwandan border. Our main 'enemy' was the FDLR (Democratic Forces for the Liberation of Rwanda), a rebel group that had among its leadership original members of the Interahamwe ethnic Hutu paramilitary group that had instigated the Rwandan genocide in 1994, killing close on a million people. Driven out at gunpoint from their home country, they were now based in the DRC where they terrorised local villages, raping and pillaging at will, setting up illegal roadblocks to extort money as well as running unlicensed gold, tin and diamond mines. It was mayhem.

To make matters even more challenging, with the capital Kinshasa close on a thousand miles away, I was the man on the ground responsible for coordinating the military operations of UN brigades from Pakistan, India and Bangladesh, three nations that do not always see eye to eye. Not only that, Goma itself is a volatile city located beneath the rumbling 11,340-foot Nyiragongo volcano – which erupted while I was there – and on the shores of Lake Kivu, a vast Rift Valley stretch of water containing huge amounts of dissolved carbon dioxide under pressure that would cause an unimaginable catastrophe if it was released. Many believe it's a case of when, not if, such an explosion occurs. Fortunately, it didn't during my tour of duty.

So it was a, well, *interesting* deployment and I had a lot on my plate. As a result, I didn't pay much attention when I started tripping and stumbling more than usual and always with my right leg. I merely assumed that was due to gravel or the rocky volcanic terrain. I couldn't put my right hand into my trouser pocket but as I'm left-handed I thought the pockets were to blame. I swapped around my keys and handkerchief to access them more easily. When cleaning my teeth, my left hand would brush normally but at the same time my right hand would float independently above the taps. No matter how hard I tried, I couldn't bring it down. It seemed to have a mind of its own, which I thought was a bit odd, but not necessarily alarming.

Another prominent symptom, one that perhaps I should have paid more attention to, was that when reading a book in bed, I couldn't turn pages with my right hand. Reading is a passion of mine but again, I shrugged this off, assuming that my lack of motor skills was due to a bug bite that had left a large lump on my arm. I told myself not to worry as it would sort itself out in time. I was also a bit strung out and wept when I read the sad parts in books such as Lieutenant General Roméo Dallaire's memoir of the Rwandan genocide *Shake Hands with the Devil*. I now know that an overwrought state is also a classic symptom of Parkinson's.

The early warning signs of the condition were there, but what with disarming rampaging rebels, dealing with disorganised DRC government troops and keeping harmony among potentially incompatible UN brigades, I had enough to worry about without considering something that I believed would fix itself.

I returned home in December 2010, thin and totally exhausted, which I had put down to a rather exhilarating tour of duty. When my nephew Charles, a military doctor in training, visited, I'm not sure if he noticed anything or if Tania said something, but he ended up carrying out some basic coordination tests. He was not happy with the results. 'You really ought to see a consultant,' he said.

I nodded. Charles had not yet qualified and would not give a diagnosis. But I have huge respect for him, and if he recommended a thorough medical examination, then I would do so. It was a pivotal moment: if he hadn't said anything, I would have just carried on as normal until everything deteriorated even further – and far more rapidly. I booked an appointment with my doctor, who initially thought I'd had a stroke or a brain tumour and referred me to the neurologist at the James Cook hospital. I felt no anger, no rage when I learnt my fate. Depression, yes – deep, dark, awful despair at times – but that was something I would have to continually control.

I'm a soldier, trained for combat, but this was a fight I knew I could not win. No one could. Instead, I had to accept it and cope as best as possible under the circumstances. I decided that while Parkinson's would obviously hinder me, I would not allow it to prevent me from doing what I wanted to do, both with my life and in my job – if the Army would still keep me on, that is. I would go on living as full a life as I could. As normally as I could.

But how could I do so under such devastating circumstances? How would I cope with my central nervous system degenerating by the day? With motor skills barely able to button up a shirt or tie shoelaces?

I was soon to find out.

2

Family Tree

I come from an adventurous family, but I think many military families can say that.

My grandfather, Wilfred Deacon, had been a reserve soldier in the Royal Monmouthshire Royal Engineers (Militia) with the British Expeditionary Force in France at the outbreak of the Second World War in 1939. He was not to come back until 1946, as he was one of forty thousand British troops who did not make it to Dunkirk's beaches during the mad scramble to be evacuated by small boats – the aptly named 'Dunkirk Miracle'. Instead, he was captured by the Germans and marched across Europe to prisoner of war (POW) camps in Poland and what was then Czechoslovakia. Many died in those brutal forced marches, and I think after that horrific experience, he decided he had little option but to wait out the rest of the war as a POW.

Wilfred's wife, Effie Deacon, my grandmother, was also part of the war effort as a NAAFI (Navy, Army and Air Force Institutes) canteen lorry driver, which meant that she could get extra rations for her young son, my father. In those early war years, life was pretty dreadful. One of her brothers, a chaplain in the Royal Norfolk Regiment, was captured in Singapore and died in the notorious Changi prison administering to the sick, while the other drowned at sea when his submarine never surfaced. With two brothers dead and her husband a POW, Effie was left to fend for herself and her small boy.

She met Jack Brown, a builder who spent every evening as an Air Raid Precaution Warden, responsible for protecting civilians during Luftwaffe bombing sprees. This was dangerous work, and not just during the Battle of Britain. Life for both Effie and Jack was lived on the edge. The inevitable happened. They fell in love and moved in together – a far more familiar story in the war than people dared admit. Wilfred returned home six years later and, having survived the appalling rigours of prison camps, he was no doubt somewhat shaken to discover his wife had run off with another man. And a 'war dodger' at that! They divorced and Effie married Jack, while Wilfred later married Nell Llewelyn Jones. Nell never really took to her husband's former family – us – and consequently I never knew my grandfather well. I suspect he was never really the same after his terrible wartime experiences. He died in 1989.

Conversely, Jack was a real playboy, while Effie was a gregarious, fun-loving woman, full of laughter and joy – just like my father. They lived life to the full and made an enchanting couple. Jack also had a passion for country sports, enjoying his shooting and racing (he had horses in training), interests which he passed on to his stepson.

On the maternal side of the family, my grandmother Lucy Jones was equally adventurous and as a teenager ran off to be a governess in Portugal. This may sound mundane today, but in 1920 it was pioneering stuff. She returned to Wales several years later and caught the eye of an older man in a hotel bar where, I believe, she played the piano. He was Charles Phillips, a retired, wealthy widower from a prominent family in Newport whose uncle had been mayor during the Chartist riots, the last time local troops were deployed against their kinsmen on British soil. I suspect Lucy saw a good thing in this rich widower and grabbed him while she could. He died before my mother turned fifteen and she was devastated.

Family legend has it that my mother met my father at Chepstow Racecourse, which is rather amusing given that she didn't particularly like racing. My father was instantly smitten by Mum, one of those classic 1950s' beauties. The fact that she was the only child of a successful mini-tycoon with an annual income of a thousand pounds from the age of sixteen (equivalent to around £50,000 today) was perhaps a bonus.

Father had chosen not to complete a degree at Imperial College in London and eventually joined the Royal Artillery. He went to Sandhurst in 1946 for two years and was then posted to his regiment in Germany. At that time, the British Army were an army of occupation more than anything else, but the situation was changing fast as the Russians were increasingly becoming the main threat to the West. My mother was living at home in Newport with her mother and when Father returned in 1954, they married at Marshfield, a village in Monmouthshire.

Not long afterwards, Father was sent to Korea with the Commonwealth Brigade to fight the Chinese. Although the Korean campaign was ending, with the bulk of hard combat over, I occasionally still heard the odd whisper about some of the exciting times he and his colleagues had. It did, however, mean that he missed the birth of my elder sister, Rowena. When he returned home two years later, the bond between my mother and her daughter was exceptionally strong, not leaving much room for him.

Shortly afterwards, Father was posted with his young family to Cyprus, where the Enosis crisis was underway, with Greek Cypriots agitating to leave the British empire and becoming more and more belligerent. This had led to the formation of EOKA, a militant group responsible for the death of many British soldiers, blowing up installations and generally whipping up widespread rebellion. It turned out the leader of EOKA, Colonel George Grivas, lived just around the corner from my family in Limassol, which was a bit close for comfort.

My father's Cyprus deployment was overall rather pleasant and Mother certainly enjoyed it. It was, however, marred by a serious accident when a Turkish policeman driving on the wrong side of the road crashed into my parents' vehicle. My mother was flung headfirst through the windscreen, landing in a ditch and rushed to hospital with a severely lacerated face. Her injuries were so bad that nurses would not give her a mirror and visitors to other patients in the ward were hurriedly ushered past. To compound matters, she was pregnant with her second child, born two months prematurely and dangerously underweight. There was great concern that the baby girl would not survive so a priest was hastily summoned and she was christened with the first name that came into my mother's head – Sarah. Anyway, Sarah did survive, and only too well, while my mother recovered with little long-term damage.

Tragically, the Turkish policeman died, and although Father was not to blame, it was nevertheless a worrying time as he faced the prospect of prison for involuntary manslaughter. However, shortly afterwards, the family were all able to return to Coventry, where Father was the adjutant of a reserve regiment before going out to Germany with 19th Field Regiment, based at Minden. The Cold War was peaking, with most of the British Army stationed in North Rhine-Westphalia and West Germany now part of NATO. Mother, Rowena and Sarah went with him.

I was born on 2 December 1961 at the British military hospital in the small town of Rinteln. I'm told I caused no delivery problems and was a normal, healthy baby. I obviously knew nothing about that. Nor, it seems, did my sisters. The first they heard about my arrival was when Father was saying his prayers with them that evening and in the 'God bless' section the name Guy was added to the list of family members – along with guinea pigs, dogs, cats and other household pets.

3

High Jinks and Education

We returned to the UK in 1962, but not for long. Two years later, Father was again sent to Germany, this time to 34th Air Defence Regiment in Hilden. He was commander of one of the artillery batteries equipped with 40/70 Bofors anti-aircraft guns that formed a defensive ring of fire around the Ruhr Valley.

I was four years old and this was the first taste of living in army accommodation that I can remember. I enjoyed it immensely as there were always other kids about to play with and the properties were large with plenty of room to roam.

From there, Father's next post was Sandhurst, Berkshire, in 1967. At first we lived on Everest Road, but then moved to The Terrace, parallel to the A3 and with much smarter residences. Ours was a three-storey house and my room was at the very top. The garden was so big that I remember Father shooting pigeons where the lawn backed onto the Wish Stream.

Sandhurst was a grand place. We had a batman called Sergeant Burns and, as Father was the master of the Sandhurst beagles, one of our chores was to walk the puppies. Always in the background was the sound of the RMAS (Royal Military Academy Sandhurst) band playing or practising for parades.

The most momentous event in my life at the time was the start of my prep schooldays. It was 1970 and my parents had looked around at the various options, deciding that Tockington Manor just outside Bristol was the school for me. It was a relatively new, privately owned school that had been a hospital until Gordon Tovey bought it in 1947. I wasn't a good student as I did not write well nor listen carefully, but I did manage to become captain of the rugby team, athletics *victor ludorum*, head of house (for what that was worth) and winner of the much-coveted senior star's prize. Most impressively I managed to pass the Common Entrance exam, much to everyone's great relief, and went to Sherborne School.

Sherborne is one of the oldest and most prestigious schools in the country, but that meant little to me as I continued on my mediocre academic path. O-levels were looking to be quite challenging. Indeed, my parents had such little confidence that they were planning on taking me away after fifth form (now called year eleven), but I stunned everyone – including myself – with an A, six Bs and a C. So great was my parents' shock that my mother thought I must've cheated! Even so, they decided to keep me at Sherborne.

It's a good thing they did as it was in sixth form that I really came of age. The first term was a bit brutal, as my good friend Nick Ross broke his neck playing rugby. I was sharing a study with him so was left bereft as he was whisked away by emergency helicopter. For me, it was a Damascene moment; my best mate was in hospital with potentially life-changing injuries and I decided that I now needed to sort out my own rather aimless life. That was when I started growing up.

Fortunately, not only did Nick fully recover, but as a demonstration of my growing maturity, not only was I working harder and taking my studies more seriously, I also started doing more 'arty' things. There was method in this madness as I had noticed that boys doing stuff such as music and theatre had far better access to the girls' school. I became involved in stage management, and later, acting and singing in the school musical society, which practised in Sherborne's chapel and the famous abbey – and which, most importantly, included girls.

One girl particularly caught my eye. She was (and still is) stunningly good-looking but at that stage I feared she was out of my league. I went out of my way to woo her and it came together one evening when I was walking her home from a music practice at the abbey and chivalrously carried her cello. After struggling all the way up the hill with the bulky instrument, she seized the initiative and our relationship was sealed with a kiss.

I was on a bit of a trajectory in other ways as well. I'd been selected for the Second XV rugby team (at that stage the First XV was undefeated), had a part in *Hamlet* and had been elected to the Stick, the upper sixth school bar. Now dating a beautiful girl as well, I was considered quite a player. There were parties most weekends and, if not, there was the Stick where we were allowed to drink beer. Finally, after completing A-levels, our class had nothing to do apart from enjoying ourselves until the end of term. When not partying, I was acting in a production of the musical *Salad Days*. Although most of my friends were in the cast, playing the leading chap opposite a beautiful heroine boosted my confidence significantly. We were having such a good time that I was rather dreading leaving school, so 'Salad Days' was an apt description for those times.

Then it all went wrong. One of the joints we frequented was a nightclub of sorts called the Taps, about three miles away from the school in Milborne Port, and after a night of revelry we only got back to school at about 2 a.m. Nobody seemed to have noticed our absence and we thought we had got away with it. But a girl partying with us had got a little too drunk and was unable to find her way back to her boarding house. One of the chaps took her to his study so she could sleep it off. Her apparent absence caused panic, resulting in a widespread search. The cat was truly out of the bag and one of our group was called upon to fulfil her civic responsibilities as a prefect. She compiled a list of everyone who had been at the Taps.

The first I knew about it was at ten o'clock the following morning when we were summoned to the headmaster's office. We were called in pairs and I was marched up the stairs with my good friend Nick Hewett. We were amazed to discover that the head knew we'd been to the Taps and even more amazed that our punishment was to be what the school called 'rustication': we were not welcome back for the next year.

I went home for the summer holiday and waited somewhat apprehensively for my A-level results. Utterly astonished, I discovered I had got an A, B and C, easily exceeding everyone's expectations again. As it turned out, my rustication was not enforced. I returned to Sherborne early for the autumn term and seventh form to join the pre-season training for rugby. This time I got into the First XV, playing lock forward alongside my great friend Andrew Spink. We were unbeaten that season and, as I had played for the Second XV the previous season, I had not lost a game for two straight seasons – not due to my brilliance, I hasten to add.

A few weeks later I was on a train up to Darlington and then a minibus to Catterick Garrison in north Yorkshire. It was a move that would change my life, opening up experiences and adventures that I would not have experienced in any other career.

I had just turned nineteen.

4

Guns and Roses

For as long as I could remember, I had wanted to join the army. My father had not specifically encouraged me, but nor had he dissuaded me. He wanted me to make up my own mind and when I did, I knew he was pleased.

In 1980, joining a regiment was like joining a club – it had to want you. I was interested in joining the Queen's Dragoon Guards (QDG), a regiment in the Royal Armoured Corps founded in 1685 that has played a prominent combat role in every conflict the United Kingdom has been involved in for the past 340 years. It's a fine regiment and fortunately for me my father knew some of its officers, so I got an audience with the hierarchy. I was interviewed by Lieutenant Colonel Charles Bond, who was to be commanding officer of the QDG from 1981–2, and I remember being very nervous, trying not to spill anything when offered a cup of tea. With the approval of the colonel of the regiment, the officers and the men, I was granted a place, as long as I passed the Regular Commissions Board (RCB) selection process. Every officer has to go through the RCB to identify leadership skills, fitness and ability to make decisions under stress.

To prepare for this, I was sent to Catterick Garrison where Trooper Deacon, service no. 24540224, was placed in Cambrai

Troop. Although billed as preparation for RCB assessment, it was little more than sanctioned bullying to weed out the weak and uncommitted. It certainly served its purpose, as out of the twenty people in my intake, only six were commissioned.

When I arrived, the Royal Hussars was the training regiment and although the course lasted just ten weeks, it felt much longer. I distinctly remember that first haircut – a real rite of passage – as well as queuing up for meals in the cookhouse, washing pans and not much spare time. We drilled relentlessly, with a little bit of leadership training thrown in and lots of block-cleaning jobs. I was usually on ablution duty, which I shared with a good friend, Richard Charrington.

We became proficient in handling SMGs (submachine guns) and SLRs (self-loading rifles) and our first exercise was on the North Yorkshire Dales. It was in the depths of winter, and just in case the unrelenting rain was not pelting strongly enough, we had to ford the frigid River Swale and were soaked to the bone and shivering before setting up a patrol base in a quarry. That night we were 'bumped' by our trainers posing as the enemy and had to retreat in disarray to a prearranged rendezvous. My first night on exercise as a paid soldier was spent hugging a stone wall for what limited shelter I could get.

Next morning, we had a kit inspection and the directing staff were merciless. We had to pay for anything left behind, lost or not properly cleaned. The staff had actually stolen some of our kit or deliberately smashed it up, but it was a strong message to hammer home the soldier's most basic code – always look after one's kit. It's something we would never forget.

Our final exercise was at Otterburn Training Estate on the Scottish border where we continued to be treated harshly. By now we were looking forward to leaving. One chap had rocks thrown at him after displaying the map indicating our route, and on another occasion we had to run to the top of a steep hill to find fictitious rubbish theoretically left behind, followed by washing in the freezing river. We also did the Lyke Wake walk, a challenging forty-mile hike in snow following an old coffin route across the highest part of the North York Moors.

It was during this period that Durham University called me up for an interview. Before joining the Army, my father had suggested I apply to Cambridge on the strength of my A-level results – not bad for someone who most thought would fail fifth form. I had no real concept of university and was advised to go to Cambridge and look at Magdalen College. A mistake as it turned out. Magdalen had been known for being a corduroy, all-male college (ideal for me) but was going through a mini-revolution to shed its traditional stuffiness. Even if I had been a strong candidate they would probably not have welcomed yet another public schoolboy. On top of that, I didn't really know what to study, so chose joint archaeology and anthropology as that was what my brother-in-law Julian was reading. During the interview I shared my non-existent knowledge of those topics, which took all of ten seconds. I was not offered a place.

Fortunately, I also had Durham University on my selection form and now they wanted to interview me. I hired a car and sped off to meet the then-famous Rosemary Cramp and Professor Sunderland from the archaeology and anthropology departments. To my delight, I not only secured a place, but it would be at the famed University College, where the castle is the oldest building in use at any university in the world. All I had to do now was pass the RCB. Thanks to the hard training at Catterick Garrison, I was quite well prepared and didn't find the process to be much of a struggle. In fact, my presentation talk was on amateur dramatics, something I had done at school. Not only did the Army agree to defer my posting by three years to complete university, they also said they would pay me nine hundred pounds a year as a bursar.

Little did I know I was about to embark on the best time of my life to date, consisting mainly of womanising, boozing, rowing and not much studying, which I think is the hallmark of most first-year university students. Of particular significance was my first night while queuing for supper when I spotted someone I thought to be an old school friend and went over to say hello. I tapped him on the shoulder, only to discover he was a complete stranger.

'Sorry, I thought you were someone else,' I muttered, slightly embarrassed.

'I'm Andrew Hartley,' he said.

He seemed to be a nice chap so I invited him to our table. The main topic every new student talked about in those initial weeks was what they had done in their gap year. I had travelled around the USA and Canada, thinking that was brave and daring, but it was nothing compared to Andrew. He had travelled overland from the UK to Australia, boating around Iran and Pakistan and then through India. He returned home via Kenya, where he made his way to Lake Turkana, a vast Rift Valley stretch of alkaline water in the middle of a desert and about as far off the beaten track as one could get. He said it was something he planned to do again.

I was intrigued. I had always wanted to travel and explore Africa, a dream inspired by a Wexas travel guide book I received as a young boy. And now someone I had just met had not only done that, but was talking about doing it again. That sowed the seed of what would be called the South Turkana Expedition and, in the course of planning the trip, Andrew became a lifelong friend.

We needed a reason for the expedition to get sponsorship. Andrew was an archaeological student, I was studying anthropology and we came up with the idea to do an updated report on the material culture of the Turkana tribe and compare it to a study compiled in 1968 by an earlier Royal Geographical Society (RGS) excursion. We recruited two geography students, David Simonson and Nick Lambert, who planned to do their dissertation on the Lake Turkana region. Andrew, who is a brilliant organiser, would be expedition leader, with me as treasurer and we managed to secure grants from both the RGS and Durham University as well as sponsorship of a Land Rover, beer, clothing and car batteries.

We flew out on Sudan Airways, the cheapest flight at the time, collected the Land Rover and loaded up our kit, including a large sack of 'tombacco', a blend of tobacco central to Turkana culture and a crucial bartering tool to get introductions to tribal leaders. After almost rolling the overloaded vehicle, we first stopped in the town of Kitale near the Ugandan border. It's a pretty rough place with a large, rundown hotel as well as a still-functioning polo club, no doubt a throwback to the pioneering settler days. Nick and David went to bed early, while true to form, Andrew and I did not. We found a bar serving ice-cold Tusker beer and settled down for the night.

We were getting on famously with the other patrons, when suddenly a bloke brandishing a machete stormed over and wanted to cause some grievous bodily harm to a chap we were talking to. From what I could gather, our 'friend' had been misbehaving with the machete man's wife, who was not happy. Trying to dodge machete blows, the alleged adulterer pleaded with us to help him. There seemed little we could do, but before I knew it, Andrew was nowhere to be seen and I was left alone with very few options. I was not the object of the assailant's wrath, I was bigger than him, probably stronger too, and I wasn't drunk. I rushed him and knocked him flat. In no time I had him pinned down with one knee on his throat and the other on his machete-wielding arm. Andrew, realising he had left me behind, bravely returned to find me shouting for assistance, which he sought from a group of passing soldiers. They took hold of the man and pacified him, at which point we beat a hasty retreat. It was a bit of a hairy moment, but we were young and believed we were bombproof, so thought it was rather funny.

The next day we continued the journey along the poorly paved north road, descending the steep Marich Pass down the Rift Escarpment towards the Turkana settlement of Lokori, which would be our base for the next eight weeks. Our first attempt at setting up camp was bang in the middle of a goat track, so we hastily moved next to a volcanic outcrop to avoid further livestock traffic jams.

We had chosen Lokori on the River Kerio as that was the site of the previous RGS survey. It was also the most convenient spot, as the Turkana are nomadic and have almost no permanent buildings. Instead, they live in *awis*, stick huts that can easily be disassembled and piled onto a camel for the next journey. They're the largest tribe in the area and as cattle rustling was part of their nomadic way of life, they weren't very popular. In fact, the whole area at the time was fraught with ancient tribal tensions; there were also cattle raiders coming across the border from Ethiopia and gangs of Somali *shifta* (bandits). It was a rough neighbourhood, but we had little inkling of that. On the contrary, we were treated amazingly well by the local people and accorded respect we didn't deserve. It was an extraordinary privilege to be so included in the local way of life and immerse ourselves in the quintessential soul of such wild country.

We got supplies from nearby Somali *dukas* (shops), but soon ran out of cash and had to get to a bank quickly. This could only be done in Nairobi, so I drove Andrew to Kitale where he caught a bus to the Kenyan capital. It was exceptionally bad timing as almost at that exact moment the Kenyan Air Force decided that President Daniel arap Moi had to go and staged a coup d'état.

The rebels' first move was to seize the national radio station and Nairobi erupted in total chaos. Andrew managed to make his way to the British embassy, avoiding the anarchy in the streets, while I decided our best plan was to flee to Ethiopia. I filled up our spare jerry cans with fuel in Kitale, then drove two hours north to our base camp to fetch Nick and David. We learned that the coup was over and the rebels defeated, but not before about two hundred people had been killed. Fortunately, Andrew was not one of them and arrived back after a week with some gruesome stories of people chopping each other up.

He also brought a bottle of whisky with him, which was much appreciated.

I am not quite sure what got into me that evening, but the bottle did not last very long at all. As we regaled each other with stories, I failed to notice that the others were drinking very little. It may have been the heat or the mosquitoes or just possibly the relief that Andrew was back in one piece but, judging by my condition the next morning, it could only have been me who was responsible for the empty bottle. I was good for nothing, so spent the bulk of the day staked out in the river allowing the water to soothe my aching head and cool my incapacitated body.

It was an extremely successful trip and our reports were well received. But even better, it was an unimaginably rich experience, exploring Africa as exuberant twenty-one-year-olds and fending for ourselves in conditions few westerners would ever encounter. It certainly gave me a taste for expeditions into wild areas. I wanted more of the same.

I didn't have to wait long. This time it would be in Algeria.

5

Dunes and a Degree

By some quirk of fate, I was appointed captain of the College Boats Club in my second year at university. Given my relative inexperience as a rower it was an unexpected accolade and I took it seriously.

Rowing therefore occupied most of my spare time, either as a coach on the towpath, or occasionally as a cox. This was unusual, as a cox is usually the smallest, lightest person on the boat and I was a rugby lock forward. So here I will let you in on a little secret; rowing is not difficult. Technique is terribly important, of course, but it's more about fitness, strength and willpower. It was not beyond my abilities by any stretch of the imagination.

We were a reasonably successful club and although we did not collect much silverware, we had a lot of fun both on and off the water. Among our more memorable events was competing in the Head of the River Race for the first time in many years, an elite against-the-clock contest on the Thames which is always raced on an ebb tide, unlike the more famous Cambridge and Oxford boat race.

Through rowing connections, as well as being expedition advisor on the Durham University Exploration Society committee, I heard that fellow student Adam Spowers was planning to lead a motorised expedition across the Grand Erg Occidental, a 60,000-square-mile swathe of Saharan desert dunes in south-west Algeria. It was to be called GEO 84, and Adam was recruiting his team from Grey College where he was an undergraduate. Luckily for me, he made an exception and it was a great privilege to be chosen as the only outsider.

Although the Erg had been crossed by camels, a motorised attempt in 1981 by an army expedition in three Land Rovers only managed to get eighteen miles before realising the enormity of the task and turning back. It was one of the last remaining challenges in desert exploration and as gung-ho students we believed that if anyone could do it, we could. This was no pipe dream. Adam, also due to join the Army, had fine leadership and organisational skills, deep technical knowledge and had been involved in two previous private expeditions to the Sahara. The rest of the team consisted of Andrew Purvis, a rower like me (but much better) who was in charge of communications; Hugh Davies, the medical officer who had been on expeditions to Tunisia and Kericho in the Kenyan Rift Valley; David Attenburrow, a physics student and mechanical genius; liaison officer Robert Stubbs, who spoke Arabic and myself. I brought along my experiences of the Turkana expedition in 1981 and also, thanks to my connections with the QDG, I could get hold of essential equipment such as tents and jerry cans. We had planned to bring along a photographer, but couldn't find someone suitable so Adam recruited his sixteen-year-old brother Rory, who would be a backup driver.

Honda agreed to lend us four off-road, three-wheeler ATVs specifically built for incredibly harsh terrain that would be our frontline vehicles, while Land Rover loaned us a brand new Range Rover to accompany Adam's old model as backup. The 'mothership' was a standard Unimog lorry carrying spares and supplies. This tough vehicle was only fitted with a two-litre engine delivering a puny 80 h.p., those wheels never stop turning.

My role initially was to drive the Unimog and I first needed to get it to Algeria to rendezvous with the rest of the team. They were at the only hotel in a one-camel town called Timimoun on the edge of the Grand Erg. Accompanied by Robert Stubbs, I caught a ferry from Marseilles to Algiers and then drove far into the desert, arriving at the hotel early. At the scheduled rendezvous time, Robert and I ordered cold beers to wash away the dust, thinking how crazy it would be for everyone actually to pitch up on time in such a far-flung location.

Half an hour later, as I was about to give up, I spotted a Range Rover in the distance coming towards me. Adam and the rest of the expedition arrived. The show was now on the road – literally. We soon discovered that the Honda three-wheelers were perfect for the job. In fact, they were so capable that they didn't really need backup vehicles as the crossing team – Robert, Hugh, Andrew and David – could pull trailers we had specifically made to hold crucial equipment and food. Consequently, we revised our plans and set about crossing the Erg in two teams from different start points: the northern section was negotiable by the Unimog and Range Rovers, while the southern part – with treacherously shifting sands – would be crossed by the tri-wheeler ATV team. We would meet in the middle.

To navigate we used Walker satnavs, state-of-the-art technology in those days but designed for maritime use, so that too was a 'first' in the desert. As with everything, simplicity worked best and the final rendezvous was marked by setting alight tyres found along the roadside producing thick black smoke that could be seen for miles.

It was a magical time of vast emptiness, hot horizons and shimmering oases. Looking out across what seemed to be infinity, as the sun set over a sand sea of beautifully sculpted dunes, as if carved by the hand of God, was something I will always savour. To this day, I prefer deserts to any other environment. It was hard going, but I cherished every minute of it. I still have photos of the Unimog careering wildly off dunes with all four wheels in the air, and the drivers of the three-wheelers taking gut-swooping spills on almost vertical slopes. Technically, GEO 84 was the first motorised crossing of the Grand Erg Occidental, but it's hard to seek official recognition seeing we've never submitted a post-expedition report! We have a reunion every five years and still laugh about that.

Honda were delighted with the performance of their vehicles, as these ATVs were designed specifically for the leisure market – later in the safer four-wheel configuration – and had never been tested in such anger before. Land Rover were equally happy and, thankfully, did not look too closely at their recently new vehicle. Indeed, this expedition had accomplished cutting-edge stuff without us even knowing it. As far as we were concerned, it had been purely a fantastic adventure. A highlight of our lives.

After that adrenalin rush, I had to settle down and do some work for the final exams. I had attended most lectures despite my hectic extramural activities: there was only one lecture a day and two essays a term; it was not exactly onerous. The biggest problem was that one of the lectures was at 9 a.m., which was a shocker given that we were almost always out partying well beyond midnight. However, I had already worked out that the exam paper questions were pretty much the same every year. The wording might be different, but the essence never varied, so I did the minimum amount of work preparing answers for the most likely three questions in each exam.

Thankfully, I was right. I managed to scrape through with a rather dodgy, third-class degree in anthropology, having dropped archaeology along the way. Some may have been disappointed with such a result, but as no employer has ever asked what class degree I was awarded, it has never held me back.

It was now time to get serious. I was about to join the Army full time.

6

Parades and a Funeral

The Royal Military Academy Sandhurst (RMAS) is where officers in the British Army are trained to lead their soldiers. It's considered to be one of the best in the world and it's not just me saying that. Many other nations send their officers there.

Despite its reputation for excellence, induction was a strange process, consisting of a lot of marching, carrying loads of kit, and having haircuts. For the first six weeks we were cut off from the outside world, getting up at five each morning preparing for inspection, which was a very thorough affair as each room had to be laid out in the same way with no non-essential personal possessions. Luckily, I had a car which I used as storage for excess stuff, but more importantly it was where I kept my duvet. This meant that once I had made the perfect bed block with edges sharply squared off as demanded by the inspecting officers, I never needed to unmake it.

A big stroke of luck was that James Moberly, my good friend from Durham University, ended up four rooms down the corridor. We helped each other with various chores to make life easier, and our friendship has lasted to this day, with him joining me on the first stage of my Parkinson's African odyssey more than thirty years later.

We weren't a particularly good platoon, but not too bad either. Frankly, I was not really challenged during my time at Sandhurst and arrived there fitter than when I left. In fact, I was only seriously tested during the march and shoot run, a cross-country shooting contest, and the log run, a gruelling team event carrying a hefty tree trunk over a considerable distance. Otherwise everything else was a bit of a breeze.

However, our Sovereign's Parade graduation day – when a successful officer cadet becomes a commissioned officer – was fantastic, not least because our inspecting officer was her majesty Queen Elizabeth II. We were the first intake to carry rifles rather than the traditional swords and I felt surprisingly proud of the fact that two days previously I'd been on an exercise in the Otterburn woods in northern England covered in muck, ready to take on the Queen's enemies, and now with the same weapon I was smart as a carrot for her majesty to inspect me. It was the first time in thirty years that she had been the Sovereign's Parade inspecting officer.

One major problem with carrying rifles on parade was that our bayonets, usually a dull-grey field colour, had to glisten like burnished silver. We set about shining them with Brillo and Brasso and, frankly, were getting nowhere when I remembered that there was a metal shop just around the corner in Sandhurst village. I took my bayonet there and after about ten seconds on a polishing wheel it was transformed into a gleaming masterpiece. Overcome with guilt for illegally taking a weapon off the academy's premises, I decided to share the blame and took all of the platoon's bayonets to the shop. It cost a pound for each polishing and was such a success that the entire college followed my example.

The parade itself went off like clockwork, the drill movements were superbly synchronised and nobody fainted. The weather was a bit gusty but we all managed to keep our hats and the advance in review order was so good it made the hair on the back of our necks stand up.

My friend Nick Pope, later a three-star general, got the Queen's Medal for the best cadet, a taste of what was to come in his illustrious career, and I was his platoon sergeant on the final exercise, which makes me think I was number two in the platoon if not on the course!

We then marched up the steps of Old College and, as per custom, bid farewell to our rifles that had been our constant companions for the past forty-four weeks. Afterwards, I was one of the lucky ones to have lunch in Old College with the Queen and that evening attended the commissioning ball where we revealed our second lieutenant's pips on our squeaky-clean mess kits.

After that, arriving at my regiment was surprisingly a bit of a disappointment. New officers straight out of the academy were prime targets to be assigned extra orderly officer duties, and the QDG is no different from other cavalry regiments with its rites of passage. There were lighthearted initiation ceremonies, generally requiring the very unimaginative requirement of downing a bottle of champagne before your buddy could eat two cream crackers. We were also constantly 'bottled' – fined a bottle of champagne for minor or imagined misdemeanours – and in many cases not allowed to speak up in our defence. It was not a welcoming process for new officers, but as there were seven of us, we easily endured this petty inhospitality. I recognised it for what it was; nothing more than a combination of establishing a pecking order and testing new officers. We were after all joining a close-knit group of officers and, as with any club, we had to establish our credentials.

Then it was off to Bovington, an Army base in Dorset between Poole and Dorchester, where I was trained as a reconnaissance troop leader on Scorpion and Scimitar armoured vehicles. I was in B Squadron, with four vehicles and twelve men under my command, and like all new officers, I needed to work closely with an experienced troop sergeant. In my case, it was a man called Fred Tyler, and I made it my business to get on well with him.

Soon afterwards, the squadron was sent to Cyprus with UNFICYP (United Nations Peacekeeping Force in Cyprus), that oversaw the ceasefire following the Turkish invasion of the island in 1974. Our job was to enforce what was known as the Green Line, a demilitarised zone separating the Greeks and the Turks, and each month we rotated to a different UN contingent. We were primarily a presence on the ground and although we exercised for riots and there were some minor tensions, there was no actual fighting. Consequently, it was a pleasant deployment with leisure time spent skiing on the snow in the Troodos Mountains or behind a boat on the warm waters in the Mediterranean.

On return from Cyprus, our commanding officer Johnny O'Brien told me I was going to spend the next summer in Bovington on a gunnery course to become the Regimental Gunnery Officer, which I guessed was an accolade even though I had yet to take part in a regimental gunnery camp. Almost immediately after completing the course I, with Sergeant 'Fat Willie' Williams, ran the regimental ranges at Castlemartin in Pembrokeshire before the regiment deployed on a major exercise to test our ability to get from the UK to our Cold War positions along the inner German border near Hanover.

On returning to the UK, to my delight I was selected as second-in-command on an expedition that would take me back to Africa, the continent that had so fascinated me since childhood. The Army calls these expeditions 'Adventurous Training Exercises' and they are superb opportunities for soldiers to test themselves in arduous physical and mental situations. The stated goals, apart from having a fantastic experience, are to develop an individual's 'loyalty, team spirit, discipline, self-respect, courage, fitness, resourcefulness, determination, adaptability, good humour, initiative and leadership'. I cannot recommend them highly enough.

The instigator of this particular expedition, called 'African Eagle', was Captain Mark Joyce, a vehicle maintenance expert based at Bovington. His plan was to drive a four-tonne Bedford truck and a Land Rover across the Sahara into West Africa's tropical jungles, then veer east across Central Africa to finish in Kenya. Mark's original proposal was to go all the way to Zimbabwe in the south, but we thought that was rather extreme with our time limits.

Anthony 'Spook' Pittman and I would be joint second command. Mark knew of my university expeditions to Kenya and Algeria, while Spook had grown up in Zimbabwe, so we both had valuable African experience. We took along nine other soldiers – all 'characters' in the regiment who were top-class team players.

The Bedford was modified at Bovington Garrison under Mark's supervision: it had extra fuel tanks, the exhaust was moved to the front to allow the tanks to be fitted and coach seating was fitted for comfort. I gave some good input based on my previous expeditions, but didn't quite get our winterisation requirements right as our single canvas cover was no match for the bitterly cold heights of the Atlas Mountains. Otherwise, the truck performed brilliantly.

We arrived in Algiers after a stormy ferry crossing from Marseilles on a boat that was more rust than steel. The best meal the ship's chef could concoct in the heaving seas was couscous, accompanied by moaning from the seasick team.

The trip through Algeria was brilliant, traversing the panoramic Atlas Mountains, then into the Sahara, which I loved. After a couple of weeks of hard going we crossed over an invisible border into Niger where there was nothing but sand and more sand, but still absolutely fascinating. There, in a town called Zinder, I sampled the best ice cream I have tasted in my life – no mean feat in the desert. Next was Nigeria, where we did some vehicle maintenance, then across Cameroon and into the Central African Republic. We stopped for a couple of days in the capital Bangui, a nice francophone city, before heading east towards a town called Kembé close to the border with the Democratic Republic of the Congo which, under the dictator Mobutu Sese Seko, was then called Zaire.

The border closed on weekends, so we camped on the River Kotto, a popular tourist spot for African overland expeditions as it had an impressive hundred-foot-high double waterfall. Just above the two waterfalls was a small lake where we bathed and cleaned the vehicles. It was the dry season so the water was not high and only one of the falls was flowing.

Spook, a chap called Spud Rhys-Jones and I were lying on the banks of the lake, sunbathing, when one of the team decided to swim across to the other side. It looked fine as the waterfall was dry where we were, so there was no current. But it was a different story on the other side where the waterfall was flowing. When the swimmer got to within ten yards of the far bank the current suddenly seized and hurled him over the falls. We saw him going over and shouted but he didn't stand a chance. Spook, Spud and I then sprinted to a bridge about a hundred yards downriver.

There was no sign of our swimmer. Spud and I took the Land Rover down the river to find a spot where he might have washed up, while Spook rushed off to tell Mark. We parked the Land Rover near the water's edge and started searching. As we were doing so, several soldiers arrived looking somewhat belligerent. I tried to explain in my best French that our friend had gone over the waterfall, but they were having none of that and arrested us for trespassing on President André-Dieudonné Kolingba's personal farm. We had no idea we were on private property, let alone that of the president himself.

The soldiers impounded the Land Rover, but fortuitously a French agronomist who was working on the farm intervened. The soldiers let us go to report the tragedy, but kept the Land Rover. It was later returned and when we met up with the rest of the team, Mark had already reported the corporal's presumed drowning to the Kembé police.

Thankfully, due to the proximity of the president's farm, there was a big satellite dish and good phone communications. We contacted the regiment back in England and the French military attaché in Bangui. When Mark called on the attaché as a military courtesy several days earlier, he said if we had any problems, we must contact him.

Well, we now had a problem. A big one. Good as his word, the attaché said that once the body resurfaced, he would send out a helicopter to fly it to Bangui, from where it would be repatriated to England.

The Kembé police told us a body normally took two weeks before bloating sufficiently to resurface and so we waited. After fourteen days, it popped up by the river's edge. However, we could not simply fly it out as we were told by police that any corpse older than two days had to be buried immediately. That was the law – in that part of the tropics the dead are, for obvious reasons, buried as soon as possible. We had no option but to comply and started building a coffin from wood bought from the local mission station, while I went around looking for embalming soap, thinking it would be useful. Despite my best schoolboy French, no soap was forthcoming. So cheap aftershave had to suffice.

However, the coffin we built was far too big, requiring a large grave. Those at the gravesite covered themselves with sickly sweet aftershave or stuffed cotton wool up their noses to mask the smell of decay. By now it was dark and as gravediggers worked under the glow of a hurricane lamp, a crowd of locals gathered to watch. The scene was eerily Dickensian, with the flickering lamp highlighting the cotton wool in people's nostrils as well as the whites of the bemused villagers' eyes.

After the burial we went back to camp and held a wake in honour of our departed colleague. The conversation was laced with typical dark army humour, which is how British soldiers deal with death and tragedy. A truck of overlanders from New Zealand joined us for the evening and were horrified at what they thought was our callousness, which was the complete opposite of how we actually felt.

We dug up the grave the next morning and moved the coffin to the village football field where a French air force helicopter would pick it up. Bemused villagers who had been at the burial the night before now came to watch the 'reverse engineering' process – and I wondered what the hell they must have been thinking. From there it got even more bizarre as we drove to the sports ground in an aftershave-drenched Land Rover playing rock music on the vehicle's cassette recorder.

As a mortician sealed the body in a lead-lined coffin, the pilot invited us for a picnic lunch complete with wine, as the French military is very civilised in that regard. They flew off as we continued on the road towards Zaire.

After that awful accident the journey was fairly uneventful. The roads and river crossings in Zaire were horrific at times, but nothing the Bedford couldn't handle. A highlight was seeing the famed 'gorillas in the mist' in the Virunga Mountains at a time before it became a tourist hot spot and from there we crossed into Uganda at Kisoro.

Uganda had recently ended its own bloody civil war where President Yoweri Museveni ousted Milton Obote, but there were still child soldiers manning roadblocks. To see hostile, blank-eyed ten-year-olds with AK-47s slung over their shoulders was an especially disturbing sight. We then rounded Lake Victoria and into Kenya, leaving the Bedford and one Land Rover with the British mission in Nairobi.

It was a strange and unforgettable journey – the magnificent desert ride through the Sahara into the vast African rain forests and along Rift Valley lakes contrasting unimaginably with the haunting tragedy of a corporal drowning. The memories of such stark extremities are indelible.

And for ever will be.

7

Hot and Cold Frontlines

On my return from Africa, the regiment was again deployed to Germany on a four-year tour. I had some leave due and joined it a week later at our new base in Wolfenbüttel, a town on the East German border. In other words, we were on the Cold War frontline.

When I arrived I wasn't feeling right, shivering with bouts of fever, headaches and muscle pains that started off as a series of niggles but worsened rapidly. I thought it was merely exhaustion, as after each fever attack I invariably felt fine. I never suspected for a moment that I was showing classic malaria symptoms. I'd religiously taken antimalarial tablets while in Africa, but stupidly stopped once back in the UK, not knowing that it was absolutely vital to complete the course for it to be effective.

Fortunately, the squadron leader, Peter Holdsworth, recognised my condition for what it was and after one particularly bad bout of shakes ordered me to see the regimental doctor. It didn't take him long to diagnose a serious case of cerebral malaria, and with a temperature soaring to 41.6 C, I was rushed to the military hospital in Hanover in a siren-blazing ambulance.

After two weeks in bed and bored out of my mind I snuck out one evening to visit James Moberly, who I thought was just down the road. He was considerably further, resulting in me being absent for the matron's evening patrol, causing consternation and irritation in equal measure but also indicating that I was probably ready for release.

After leave, I returned to base in Wolfenbüttel fully recovered and ready to assume active duty. It was an interesting deployment – the threat of the Cold War turning hot was slim by the late 1980s, but it was still real and we regularly shadowed Warsaw Pact forces on our patrols. We knew that if the full might of the Soviet Union and its allies came sweeping across the Wolfenbüttel border, NATO's frontline troops in the area – in other words, us – would be overrun. We were the proverbial tripwire and trained for a worst-case scenario, in which we would hide in the countryside and report back on hostile troop movements to give the second line of NATO defence time to counter-attack. Consequently, we weren't provided with the best equipment as our chances of survival were considered to be low. But we knew what we had to do and were well prepared, able to deploy the entire regiment in under four hours. We also thoroughly scouted the area and knew exactly where we could take cover and stay in the fight if the balloon went up.

Despite the constant tension and patrols, we still managed to fit in a lot of skiing, sailing and other wonderful outdoor stuff. Fortunately, the Warsaw Pact didn't do anything silly and by 1987 US President Ronald Reagan and Mikhail Gorbachev, his Soviet counterpart, were talking to each other. But even so, few of us would have guessed that the Berlin Wall would come crashing down two years later.

So, with Armageddon averted, I started planning yet another African adventure. The idea had actually come to me while recovering from malaria, but I vowed that this time would be different, as I would be the leader.

As mentioned, I had developed quite a taste for the hard, adventurous life on safari, and luckily for me, the army encouraged such missions. However, to interest sponsors, an expedition needs a *raison d'être*, tentative or not and, while daydreaming in a hospital bed, I stumbled upon an ideal one. The following year, 1988, marked the hundredth anniversary of the 'discovery' of Lake Turkana by Count Sámuel Teleki – and what better way to celebrate this than to walk in the footsteps of the great Hungarian explorer himself? Of course, the local tribes had known about the lake since time immemorial, but Teleki was the first white person to set eyes on this massive jade-coloured 'sea' in the middle of the desert.

Teleki named it Lake Rudolf after his patron, Crown Prince Rudolf of Austria, but in 1975 it was renamed Lake Turkana after the people that lived there. I had been to the lake with Durham University's South Turkana Expedition six years previously and I knew this would be no walk in the park. On the contrary, Teleki's journey took him through some of the most challenging backcountry imaginable, including the Chalbi Desert, the Sugata Valley – a cattle rustlers' hideout much like the old Wild West Badlands – and the still-active Barrier Volcano complex.

I championed the fact that there was a regimental link to Teleki, as Rudolf's father Franz Joseph, the emperor of Austria, had been appointed colonel-in-chief of the King's Dragoon Guards by Queen Victoria in 1896. This was one of the forerunner regiments of the QDG (formed in 1959 on amalgamation with the Queen's Bays) and the emperor himself had given permission for the famous *Radetzky March* to be the official regimental march, while the imperial eagle of Austria became our cap badge.

The expedition would be called 'Teleki's Return', and I selected Lieutenant Tim Woodward as my second-in-command, a new officer in the QDG who would be responsible for raising funds and administration, with team members Dixie Dean, Eddie Eld, Ivor Morris, Dave Coulson and Trooper Karl Dakin.

The expedition was divided into two sections: first we would do the Chalbi safari from Mount Kenya to Lake Turkana by vehicle and then we'd walk from the town of Maralal to the lake, following the final stages of Teleki's route into the unknown (for Europeans at that time) as closely as possible.

The initial destination was Mount Kenya, as Teleki was the first explorer to climb the south-western slopes of Africa's second-highest mountain, although he didn't reach the summit. Climbing the 17,000-foot peak is a challenge under any circumstances and as we didn't have much time, there was no need to risk altitude sickness which would have kiboshed the entire expedition. Instead, we drove to the meteorological station at a thousand feet and then hiked for about eight hard hours – six uphill and two down. Much of the climb consisted of steep, saturated marshlands that mountaineers call 'vertical bog'. It certainly ensures sopping wet socks.

From there we drove north to Marsabit, the only town of note for many miles, and then towards Lake Turkana. *Shifta* – cattle rustlers – still sporadically operated in the area and a couple of weeks previously twenty people had been killed in clashes with bandits. Thankfully, everything had quietened down by the time we arrived, and we also visited the anthropological site of Koobi Fora on the eastern shores of the lake. This UNESCO World Heritage Site is the so-called cradle of mankind as it's where the two-million-year-old skull of a *Homo habilis* – one of the earliest hominids – was discovered in 1972, leading to a dramatic revision of evolution at the time.

The next phase of the expedition was to retrace Teleki's journey on foot through Kenya's Northern Frontier District to the banks of the lake, as he obviously had no vehicles. We set aside three weeks to complete this; a potentially tight deadline to hit, but it was imperative we arrived at Teleki's Volcano on 6 March 1988, the exact date that he reached the lake a century beforehand. We couldn't be late as we planned to meet up with the British, Austrian and Hungarian ambassadors who would be driving up from the coast.

The walk's starting point was Maralal and we camped outside Wilfred Thesiger's house. The renowned explorer and SAS veteran suffered from Parkinson's disease in his final years, but when we met him he was a sprightly, albeit eccentric, seventy-eight-year-old, and the historical motive for our expedition appealed to his pioneering spirit. It was certainly an honour to meet one of the great adventurers of the twentieth century.

Although a small market town, Maralal is the capital of Samburu County and we recruited two guides to assist us; one would provide donkeys to carry our equipment; the other knew the area well, although he had a penchant for alcohol, as we later discovered. Donkeys are extremely hardy, notoriously stubborn and slow, but we could not have done without them. However, one night we had a major scare from a roaming hyena and if the donkeys hadn't woken us up in the nick of time by stamping their feet, we would have lost them. As we scrambled out of our sleeping bags, the hyena was barely ten yards away, coolly eyeing which of the beasts of burden would be the more delectable midnight snack. We pelted the predator with stones and shone torches in its eyes until finally the donkey-handler chased the hyena away with his spear.

Another problem was that the two Kenyans were not impressed with our staple diet of spaghetti, referring to it as 'white man's worms'. As a result, they were continuously hungry until we were resupplied with more agreeable rations. Water management in such arid conditions was also crucial and, although there were various wells along the way, these were often dry or polluted. Boiling and sterilising may make water drinkable, but not necessarily palatable. Even disguising the taste with industrial-strength tea was not much of an improvement.

I was the only member of the team to walk the entire distance, which I felt I had to do as the leader. Two members were required to move the truck for each leg and I rotated that duty among the men equally. But even so, it was tough on all of us – not least our self-appointed chef, Corporal Morris. He started the expedition as a rather 'round' soldier, but by the end was a mere shadow of his former self, losing four stone.

We reached Lake Logipi four days before our deadline, but still had to cross the Barrier, an active volcanic complex that separates Lake Turkana from the Sugata Valley. It's an unrelenting, nightmarish hike through barely discernible tracks strewn with large boulders and sharp lava rocks. Even the extraordinarily tough donkeys had a tough time traversing it. We finally reached Teleki's Volcano on the south of the Barrier where we were tentatively scheduled to meet the ambassadors the next day.

However, as we were not sure whether they would be keen to climb the rocky volcano in temperatures soaring to close on 50 C, we made an alternative plan to meet at the lake's edge. It was the correct decision, as when three of us reached the cinder cone peak, no one else was in sight. We worded a message with large red stones on the side of the summit, 'Teleki's Return 1st The Queen's Dragoon Guards 1988', before descending. Perhaps it is still there.

From there it was four miles to Nubayatom, another volcano perched on the lake's bank, and this was the last – and certainly worst – part of the walk. Being fairly new by geological standards, the still-brittle lava looked like a petrified set of rapids, often snapping and causing nasty cuts if we fell. We got there at the hottest time of day and on reaching Lake Turkana we plunged fully clothed into the water, despite the fearsomely large crocodile population – both in numbers and size. Semi-crazed by thirst, we also drank the foul-tasting alkaline water that made two team members sick.

Later that day we met up with the embassy team as scheduled and presented the Austrian ambassador with a QDG plaque that we'd carried all the way for the occasion. They had planned informal centennial celebrations that night, but we were totally exhausted from the arduous trek and in no mood for a party. Instead, we decided to rest before hiking to the settlement at Loiyangalani where the expedition Bedford was waiting to take us back to Nairobi.

Meeting up with the support party at the truck was a supreme anti-climax. We'd all lost our appetites and no one wanted to drink alcohol, settling instead for a pot of tea and a pint of squash. What we craved most was a shower and sleep. After three weeks of hardy independence and self-sufficiency, the toughest test had now started – readapting to civilisation.

That trip was a milestone for me in more ways than one. It was not only a rare adventure, showing the regimental hierarchy that I was capable of leading a difficult and arduous expedition, but something else also happened. While sitting on a rocky outcrop admiring the vast wild expanse of Kenya's Northern Frontier District with nothing but a static-crackling radio for company, I decided to embark on another mission.

This time to volunteer for selection to the SAS, arguably the toughest special forces regiment in the world.

8

Failing Myself

I flew back to my regiment in Germany and immediately started getting ready for SAS selection. I now ran everywhere I could with a laden rucksack thumping on my back, preparing for probably the toughest physical challenge of my life.

Little did I know that the key challenge would instead be mental.

Soldiers can volunteer for the SAS from any branch of the military, provided they have completed three years of service and are not older than thirty-two and, as everyone knows, selection is brutal. It has to be if the SAS is to remain the elite of the elite. By far the majority of applicants fail – 90 per cent, in fact. In some years no applicants have passed. Some have died in the attempt. It's no disgrace to fail and those who do are returned to their unit with no black mark whatsoever.

Coincidentally, Lieutenant-Colonel Michael Boissard had been appointed commanding officer of the regiment and asked me to be his adjutant. Unfortunately, I had little idea of the importance of the position and, as I was dead set on joining the SAS, I turned it down. What I should've said was I was about to try for selection but if that didn't work I would be honoured to accept. How different my life would have been if I had shown a bit more diplomacy and maturity. Instead, I burnt some important bridges.

When I arrived at the SAS home in Hereford in February 1989 on a cold rainy day, I was well prepared – super fit, a good shot, I knew how to read maps and had a fair grasp of Morse code. There were twenty officers and about 150 men in my intake, but we all knew most would soon be weeded out.

The first week started off well, involving hard but manageable physical exercises in the Black Mountains, as well as learning how to handle new weapons and also a new language to keep us busy in the evenings. Although challenging, it was fun. The second week was a lot tougher with gruelling marches such as the 'Fan Dance', a fifteen-mile hike with full combat load over Pen y Fan, the highest mountain in South Wales and 'Point-to-Point', where we were rigorously tested on endurance, map reading and navigation skills. All marches were timed. It was also a bitterly cold mid-winter with volunteers now starting to drop like flies.

But that was nothing compared to the third week. It's simply known as 'Test Week' and it's hellish, consisting of daily marches with ever-increasing loads and distances. The ultimate killer was the 'Endurance March', a forty-mile slog wearing a 70-pound Bergen rucksack that has to be completed in twenty hours.

Things started to go wrong for me about halfway through Test Week. Despite having run with a heavy rucksack almost continuously while training, my back and feet started to ache almost unbearably. Perhaps my preparation had not been rigorous enough after all. What I now realise is that the instructors were playing mind games with us. For example, after a day where I thought I had done well, I was called aside and warned that I was expected to do better the next day. Bloody hell, I thought, somewhat discouraged. I'd done my best and it wasn't good enough. This warning made me take stock of the situation, as volunteers were allowed one yellow card. If my name was called out and I got a warning the next day, it would indicate I had one last chance.

That's what happened. My name was called out.

I had an hour in the back of a Bedford to mull over my situation as we were taken to the day's start point, deep in the Black Mountains. Crippling doubts started to creep into my mind, eroding what little self-confidence I now had. If I had given it my best shot the day before and that was not good enough, how was I going to survive the remaining days, which were going to be even tougher? Failure seemed inevitable so I decided I may as well jack it in now and avoid the increasing pain which came with each day. I told the instructor who was running the staggered starts that I was giving up.

He looked at me hard. 'Go to the side and have a good think about it.'

I shook my head. I had already buckled so stuck to my decision. It was the first failure of my career.

There's no doubt that SAS selection is a gruelling physical test, but it's even more of a psychological test. What the selectors wanted to find out was how far I was prepared to mentally push myself through barriers of extreme physical stress. By goading me, saying they expected better, they wanted me to prove I was not going to give up. They wanted me to hoist two fingers and say, 'You won't break me.' If I had shown that resolve, they possibly would have selected me even if I had been the slowest person in the group – which I wasn't.

I'd clearly failed that test. I'm not saying I would have passed otherwise, but I certainly failed myself.

What I know now is that although fitness, strength, courage and other attributes are vital for selection, the SAS is looking for something extra. They're looking for people with a ruthless determination to succeed at any cost. Men who can physically push themselves to the absolute limit, but also have the mental ability to carry out extremely dangerous operations – and still kill the king's enemies. That's why those who pass are often not the most likely candidates on paper. For example, one volunteer in my intake whom I knew well from Sandhurst arrived with little training and was regarded as the black sheep of his regiment. Yet he had mastered mind over matter to such an extent that he breezed through the course.

And that's what the selection test is all about – to find such people. That's why SAS soldiers are the best in the world.

Only three officers out of the twenty who started with me passed selection. But pass or fail, I believe any soldier in the British Army worth his salt should try out for the SAS. That course was a profound experience. I learnt something invaluable and I learnt it in the hardest way possible. Never, ever talk yourself down.

It's something I have not forgotten and has helped significantly in coping with Parkinson's – a disease which specialises in making one feel worthless.

I am indeed indebted to the SAS in that regard.

9

Posted to Paradise

After three weeks at Hereford, I returned to the regiment. Having turned down the adjutant's position, the Army had to find something else for me to do. I had no option but to take whatever came my way.

What happened next was far better than I expected. It was a posting to a tiny Central American country called Belize. Ironically, that's probably where I would have been sent for advanced jungle training if I had passed SAS selection. Belize lies just south of Mexico and is more like a Caribbean island than the rest of the Central American isthmus. As a former British colony, it's the only English-speaking nation in the Hispanic subregion so its ties with anglophone Caribbean countries such as Jamaica are far stronger than with its mainland neighbours. It also has the archetypal laidback, island-in-the-sun attitude, which is rather pleasant. In other words, it dances more to Bob Marley than the Gipsy Kings.

Initially colonised as a foothold to contest Spanish economic interests in the eighteenth century, Belize got its independence in 1973. This immediately resulted in a bitter border dispute with Guatemala, who threatened to invade the pint-sized country. The Belizeans, seriously out-gunned and out-numbered, asked for British help, and that, in a nutshell, was why we were there.

Britain was also committed to training the Belize Defence Force, which at the time consisted of a battalion, two patrol boats – one of which was always out of service – and two Islander aircraft. However, the British contingent was a formidable force; a well-trained battalion supported by half a field battery of 105 light Howitzers, two troops of Scorpions, six helicopters, four Harrier jump jets, as well as a Royal Navy West Indies Guard Ship and SAS troops doing jungle warfare exercises. I was there as one of the captains supporting the regiment in the field, which happened to be the Royal Gurkha Rifles when I arrived, followed by the Welsh Guards and Royal Highland Fusiliers during my second deployment. Our commander, Brigadier Dick Lamb, was a fine man who gave us free reign to play hard as long as we worked hard.

Which we did.

However, as it was unlikely that the Guatemalans would attack us, there was plenty of entertainment on our time off. I was about to have the most wonderful time in my military career. Belize City, where we were based at Airport Camp, was little more than a big town boasting restaurants – where the dish of the day varied from beans and chicken to chicken and beans – and some extremely dodgy bars. Nightlife centred around Legends, a club that served great Cuba libres, and Raoul's Rose Garden, a bar two hundred yards down the road from our base catering for soldiers in more ways than one. Doctors regularly monitored the girls.

But it was the outdoor entertainment that made life so enjoyable. The beaches were spectacular, as one would expect in a garden of Eden and much of our leisure time was spent cruising in water taxis to the outlying cays, palm-fringed reef islands surrounded by turquoise waters. This led to me doing a scuba course at St George's Cay and I became a diving enthusiast. The magnificent Belize Barrier Reef is the second-largest coral reef in the world, and thanks to the Army, I explored much of it.

Apart from the beaches, I spent many weekends going deep into the beautiful rainforests with my old university friend Adam Spowers. I was going to be replacing Adam, but having failed SAS selection, I arrived early and we had the chance to do some exploring together. This was exciting stuff as most of the rainforest roads were ankle-deep mud baths, a complete contrast to the vast sand dunes that Adam and I had traversed in the first motorised crossing of the Grand Erg Occidental nine years earlier.

The Belize jungle has incredible wildlife, with a healthy population of jaguars and tapirs – not to mention venomous snakes – and, in the course of being responsible for conservation in addition to my other duties, I met an extraordinary American biologist called Sharon Matola. She was born in Baltimore and enlisted in the United States Air Force where she received jungle training. After leaving, she graduated in biology at the New College of Florida and, with few job prospects, joined the Circus Hall of Fame as an assistant lion tamer. She also later worked as an exotic nightclub dancer in Mexico to fund her day job doing biological field work.

This – the field work, not the dancing – attracted the attention of filmmaker Richard Foster, who hired her in 1982 to care for animals he was using in the making of a wildlife documentary in Belize. When the film was completed, the animals were basically abandoned as they were so habituated to humans they could not be released back into the wild. On a whim, Sharon decided to care for the animals herself and started the Belize Zoo and Tropical Education Centre. This initially consisted of some ramshackle cages and her first visitors were patrons from a nearby restaurant. To the British Army's credit, among her early supporters were soldiers doing jungle training who dug paths and renovated animal enclosures in their spare time. Sharon never forgot that.

A breakthrough was being hired as the animal consultant for *The Mosquito Coast*, filmed in Belize. Sharon so impressed the star actor, Harrison Ford, that he became one of the zoo's staunchest supporters. She then became known as the 'Jane Goodall of jaguars', after the British expert on chimpanzees, and her zoo – which only took in injured or orphaned animals – was globally recognised.

Sharon was a larger-than-life character and I spent memorable times chilling out with her, drinking beer and having a lot of laughs at the zoo. She died from a heart attack in 2021 at the relatively young age of sixty-six, but her superlative legacy lives on. Today the Belize Zoo hosts 125 native species.

Another of my duties was coordinating and preparing for disaster relief, as Belize faces directly into the hurricane belt. And sure enough, at the end of my first six-month stint in September 1989 Hurricane Hugo came blasting across the Caribbean towards us. Although it missed Belize, veering north towards the Gulf of Mexico, it hit Montserrat with a vengeance. Ninety per cent of homes on the small island suffered serious or total roof loss.

Montserrat is a British Overseas Territory, and as the nearest British military base, we were best placed to provide help. I flew to nearby Antigua with a signals team and troop of Royal Engineers as the RAF decided the Hercules transport plane was too big to land at Montserrat's airport. From Antigua I hitched a lift to Plymouth, the beleaguered island's capital, on the helicopter provided by HMS *Alacrity*, the West Indies Guard Ship at the time.

On arrival, it was clear that the Royal Navy had things under control. I wasn't quite sure what more I could do, but while walking around Plymouth I bumped into a CNN reporter who promptly interviewed me. Although trained as an Army publicity officer, I didn't expect to be appearing on global television and I had to shoot from the hip with my knowledge of hurricanes. Anyway, my grandmother saw the interview and thought I achieved that aim.

While on Montserrat, I watched in awe as a 98-foot Canadian air force Hercules landed on the short Plymouth airstrip, literally using every inch of the short runway. Not to be outdone, the RAF decided they could also do that and I remained on the island to coordinate aerial relief efforts. I spent the first night on HMS *Alacrity*, where officers dressed for dinner just as they would in England and I got into a bit of trouble when I unwittingly broke protocol after a few beers and sat in the wrong chair. As the RAF crew flew back each night to their four-star hotel in Antigua, I moved to the Royal Engineers' campsite in Plymouth where I was provided with a well-worn camp bed. I suppose that's a snapshot of how different the service branches are even though we're all part of the same team; the navy happy with their wardrooms; the RAF happy with their hotel and the engineers happy with their tents.

I was ordered back to Belize after a week as Princess Anne, who, as colonel-in-chief of the Corps of Royal Signals, was about to visit Belize and I was her designated publicity officer. I flew into Miami airport, feeling very conspicuous in an Army uniform in a foreign country and then to Belize to meet up with my fellow captain, Barry Keegan, just before the Princess Royal arrived. Little did Barry and I know that her separation from her husband Mark Phillips – a former Queen's Dragoon Guards officer – was to be announced that evening. When we heard, we were sure that she was in Belize primarily to evade the hordes of British reporters, as the seven-hour time zone difference would be out of sync with tabloid deadlines. It worked to some extent, as the press corps camping outside our gates was small by British standards, although still like pit bulls. My job was to shield the Princess Royal, so I deliberately gave straight press conferences without comments on her personal life and certainly didn't talk about anything I knew nothing about. I think I did a good job, as before she left, she thanked me for keeping the press at arm's length and also for the work I did that overlapped with her regiment. Finally, she gave me an autographed photograph, which I still have.

Shortly after that I returned to the UK for my junior staff course at Warminster, which every captain in the Army has to do. I had been doing a staff job at Belize without proper training, which was now being rectified. While there, the Berlin Wall came tumbling down. I was watching it on television in the officers' mess hall and it struck me that, as the Queen's Dragoon Guards were so heavily involved in Germany, and always had been, life was about to change significantly. Our main task for the past several decades had been guarding the inner German border, but after the iron curtain collapse, it no longer existed. Effectively, we were out of a job – although that didn't last for long, thanks to the ever-turbulent Middle East. '*C'est la guerre,*' as the French say.

After passing the junior staff course, I returned to Belize for my second six-month tour and it was as good, if not better, than the first one. I teamed up with Paul Denning, a Royal Marine whom I had met on the course and we spent much of our spare time gadding about on road trips rather than hanging out at the regular Army haunts at Airport Camp. We could do this as I had a Jeep, one of the few army personnel to have a private car, which meant I was deliberately independent and could go places where other people could not. Belize was truly my home from home.

However, while I was having the time of my life in August 1990, Iraqi president Saddam Hussein invaded Kuwait and Britain committed a division that included most of the Queen's Dragoon Guards to retake the oil-rich emirate. But as I was in Belize, I was not available for deployment.

Every combat soldier wants to be tested on a battlefield, and I was no exception, waiting anxiously for a call to join the regiment in the Middle East. But to my dismay, I missed out when plans for me to relieve a fellow officer who was due to do his staff course were denied by divisional headquarters. Consequently, on leaving Belize I was almost immediately sent to Mauritius on a short-term stint training their Special Mobile

Force. Mauritius was briefly a British colony. It is still part of the Commonwealth and we trained their police who are responsible for military functions as well as law enforcement.

It all sounded wonderful – another tropical paradise posting on palm tree beaches. But having spent a year in an even better tropical paradise, I was now missing home. However, I had no option and after just a day in England I travelled to Port Louis, the island capital.

Although Mauritius lived up to its reputation as an Indian Ocean Eden, I remember it most for being a catalogue of women problems. Through little fault of my own, I hasten to add. My previous track record was not bad – unlike today I could dance, tell amusing tales and had no problem finding a dancing partner. I aimed very high and up until this time had had three serious girlfriends, all of whom had me spellbound. In each case I could not believe my luck and in each case, I was smitten. But coins have two sides and as each ended, I was left emotionally drained and in tatters. Despite a lot of water passing under the bridge, each still holds a special place in my heart. But I could not afford the bruising that followed, so was determined to play my cards differently in future. Which did not work really either, making Mauritius much more complicated than it should have been.

It began with Brigitta, a striking German woman I was trying to date, but just as I started making some headway, two girls came out from England to visit me. Unbeknown to them, I'd had a previous fling with both, but luckily my grace-and-favour bungalow had four bedrooms, so the situation was manageable if a bit uncomfortable. Brigitta was not impressed.

Then, completely to my surprise, a colleague's girlfriend arrived and occupied another room in the bungalow. She assured me she was his ex-girlfriend and her arrival created some tension in the house – and outside, impressing Brigitta even less. Then, with accommodation getting a bit tight, an ex-girlfriend of mine arrived, bringing her new boyfriend who promptly proposed to her (and she said, 'Yes') adding to the complications.

Finally, as if nothing could get worse, a fellow officer arrived with his wife, and it was soon obvious that she was not at all happily married. I wisely kept my distance, although the officer thought otherwise, culminating in a rather awkward showdown. And with that, Brigitta scarpered.

Mauritius had been an interesting posting, if perhaps not quite in the way I hoped. I would have been quite happy with the island's other attractions, such as dodos and pink pigeons – and things would certainly have been much simpler.

10

Crisis in Kuwait

After the Mauritius deployment, I returned to the regiment in Germany. Or what was left of it. Our barracks was like a ghost town with almost everyone in Saudi Arabia about to advance into Kuwait. With no one around or any kit to look after, there was not much to do.

As it turned out, the First Gulf War lasted a mere hundred hours and was a bit of a damp squib as far as combat soldiers were concerned. The regiment was soon on its way back from Iraq and I was there to meet the flotilla of buses as they arrived at the Wolfenbüttel base. The casualty list was mercifully low, with fifteen people killed – three by the enemy, four in road accidents and eight by the Americans. However, they all had medals, and the Army is all about having medals.

I hung around for a week or two before being sent back to the UK to do a sub-unit commander's tactical course to prepare me to be a squadron leader. Three days later I got a call from Germany saying the Army was looking for people to go to Kuwait as part of the UN Iraq–Kuwait Observation Mission (UNIKOM) and, having missed out on the hundred-hour war, I immediately volunteered. Although it wasn't a combat role, it would at the very least take me to the desert which I loved. It was also part of my desire to make the most of every exotic posting available.

I was selected along with nineteen other people to join the British contribution. Our main role was to make sure the Iraqis remained in Iraq. However, given the rapid formation of the mission, the UN hadn't had time to think through all the practicalities of establishing a 158-mile demilitarised zone. All we knew was that we were going to Kuwait to provide an observer team along the border and the fundamentals of doing so would be worked out on arrival. That might sound a little haphazard, but on the credit side it allowed me to write my own rule book for the mission simply because there *was* no rule book.

We arrived to an unimaginable hell. Looking out of the windows of the Hercules flying us into Kuwait, all I could see was burning oil derricks. The black smoke strangling the desert was so thick it was like night. We landed in what I thought to be drizzle, but was actually fine droplets of oil, covering everything in a greasy film. As the Iraqi Army had retreated from Kuwait, Saddam Hussein instructed his officers to torch every oil well they could. International firefighters such as Red Adair were called in to quell the flames scorching the sky for as far as the eye could see.

I became UNIKOM's intelligence officer and my job was to identify the positions of the original Iraq and Kuwait border posts, which we could only guess at thanks to the skimpy information available. I was provided with a Land Cruiser and with the broad definitions of my job allowing freedoms that can only otherwise be dreamt about, I spent three months crossing the desert, often on my own, marking various map coordinates. I loved it. I was a real man of independence. As long as I produced results, of course.

The next three months were radically different, as the UN decided I was having too good a time by myself and I should be doing more mundane jobs at the actual observation posts. Then it went pear-shaped. Apparently, civilians – mainly farmers and their families living close to the border – were instructed by the Iraqi authorities to dig up the thousands of anti-tank and personnel mines that had been laid to deter the Allied army's blitzkrieg advance. Saddam's army no doubt wanted to reuse them as, for the Iraqis, this war was not over.

The results were predictably and brutally tragic. Civilians, including women and children, suddenly started arriving at UN observation posts with terrible injuries, ranging from shrapnel wounds to severed limbs or even loss of life. Overnight, our posts were transformed into emergency clinics with no preparation whatsoever. My rudimentary first aid techniques improved exponentially and for the next two weeks a basic camp bed was our blood-soaked operating table where, with limited experience, we tried to perform miracles to keep victims alive until they could be airlifted to hospitals.

After six months I'd had enough, and in any event, the UN decided that there were too many British and American members on the team and reduced us from twenty to seven personnel. My tour was over and it was a great relief to fly home. Although tired and worn out, I now had plenty of leave due and good money in my pocket as UNIKOM paid us an extra $207 a day – phenomenally huge in those days. I went to stay with my parents in Amesbury, Wiltshire, before renting a thatched cottage in the Test Valley that belonged to a chap who loved chalk-stream fishing. This started a passion for fly fishing as I found concentrating on delicately casting a fly cleanses one's mind. One of the cruelties of Parkinson's is I cannot fly fish anymore.

Then out of the blue I got an invitation to attend a wedding in Cheshire almost two hundred miles away. It was going to change my life.

11

Tania

Initially I was not keen on going to the wedding. Not only was Cheshire about a two-hundred-mile drive north, but I barely knew the bridal couple. The link was that the bride's mother was my godmother, but even that was tenuous as I hadn't seen her for a long time. Yet both she and my mother were insistent on my attendance.

In my opinion, the only benefit for someone like me going to a wedding is that it's sometimes a good place to meet single women. I accepted, thinking that if the worst came to the worst I might still meet someone interesting. In 1992 many of my friends were getting hitched. In fact, they were falling like ninepins – if my memory is correct, at least six got married that year – whereas I was not only single, but didn't even have a serious girlfriend. I suppose my guard was up as I had been emotionally burnt in those three previous relationships, all very intense and each with beautiful women, so was not looking for another.

Even more surprising than my wedding invitation was that I was placed at the top table with the bride and groom, Caroline and Henry Wilkinson. Why had I, an outsider, been accorded this honour? The answer was sitting right next to me. Her name was Tania and she had been strategically placed by my godmother who thought I would be the right man for her. Tania was friends with the bride's family and knew more than I did about the seating arrangements, although not much, and was clearly somewhat embarrassed by the whole process.

We got chatting and she told me she had just got back from Hawaii where she had been a windsurfing instructor. I was impressed. Who would have thought that an English rose would be teaching brawny islanders how to windsurf at some of the world's most iconic big-wave beaches? She struck me as being a gutsy person and certainly very athletic. I could see right away that she was competitive and ambitious – two qualities I didn't have in abundance at the time. Although that was changing as now being a squadron leader, I was starting to realise my own military potential.

After the reception we adjourned to a nearby pub. She told me she lived in Romsey, Hampshire, which was not far from Tidworth Camp where I was based, so it was not much of a struggle to agree to meet again. Things started slowly, not least because she went off to Canada for the winter to ski in the Rockies when, much to my surprise, I found myself looking forward to seeing her again.

One thing led to another, and we started dating about two weeks after her return. Being sporty, she often cycled on her mountain bike to my cottage in Amport and that was something else I found attractive about her. She did not fit the stereotype of an officer's wife or girlfriend.

Our romance was on a slow burn. Unlike some couples, we didn't have to be together the whole time. She again flew off to Canada not long afterwards for the next big mountain skiing season. She's world-class on the steepest black runs and her being away gave me a bit of breathing space to polish my own meagre skiing skills with friends in the Alps. I also bought myself a windsurfer. I obviously couldn't keep up with her in either sport, but I wanted at least to hold my own. She was brilliant at whatever she did and I was in awe of that.

Tania didn't particularly relish army life and I never made a big deal out of it. I was attending staff college at the time, the flagship academic course that an officer had to attend to make the highest ranks in the Army. I was living in the splendour of the Victorian staff college building which was dripping in history and I was surrounded by the brightest officers of my generation. My course was exceptional and produced one full general, seven lieutenant generals, three major generals and a staggering twenty brigadiers. I was in very good company and the course record has never been bettered.

As I lived in the college, I was in the parish of the Royal Memorial Chapel, where the pillars are adorned with the names of officers who fell in the First World War and I was eligible to get married there. Not only was it a wonderful building for such a ceremony, but the staff college was also a fitting venue for the reception. And it had the added advantage of allowing us to organise our wedding rather than rely upon our parents (Tania's being bitterly divorced). It was a winter wedding: she wore velvet and our honeymoon was spent in Andalusia, where we planned to go skiing. It was great – except with one flaw: no snow fell in southern Spain that year.

My first posting as a married man was in Bovington and it was a highlight of our early married life. We lived in Foxbury Road where our neighbours were all newly-weds and it was one long party for two years, with plenty of outdoor pursuits such as shooting, fishing, skiing and swimming in the sea. Tania and I still have good friends from that time. Our house was so close to the barracks that I walked to work, while Tania carried on with her successful marketing career.

Then misfortune struck. At the end of our second year of marriage, Tania fell pregnant but miscarried. It was a time of sorrow and Tania had to further adjust as we were moving out of Dorset to Sennelager in Germany.

It was easy for me as I'd been appointed squadron leader of my old unit, B Squadron. Now on tanks, previously I had been a reconnaissance squadron leader, which is more of a coordination role, stuck in a mobile office collating reports from the troops closest to the action. A tank squadron leader, on the other hand, is a commander in his own right, leading a squadron of twelve tanks from the front and hitting the enemy as hard and fast as possible in much the same way that the cavalry had in times gone by. There is nothing more exciting than a well-drilled squadron charging with infantry and supported by artillery into an enemy position and destroying it – even though they were practice sessions. The squadron was good at it, and so was I.

However, Tania hated being far away from home and her dogs. She was not ready for a life where everything revolved around the army and the fault is mine as I didn't prepare her for it. The intense military environment of Sennelager was a far cry from the freewheeling lifestyle we had at Bovington and she had been thrown into the deep end. To add to the stress, I also travelled a lot, including two training tours at the British Army Training Unit Suffield (BATUS) in Canada and a tour of Northern Ireland.

Thankfully for her sanity and our marriage, halfway through my tour, the regiment moved back to England, this time to Catterick in Yorkshire. We relocated to much better army quarters, collected our dogs and she was far happier, now mingling with other like-minded people. Our son Wilfred was born as we left Germany and Tania got to know other military mums in similar situations. North Yorkshire had the added advantage of excellent field sports, which we both loved.

Soon afterwards, I was again sent to Canada. BATUS is seven times the size of the Salisbury Plain Training Area and this massive Canadian prairie in Alberta was the make-or-break test for tank people. All exercises involved live munitions, something we could never do in tiny Britain and everything was rigorously assessed. The consensus was that if you did well at BATUS, you were set for the rest of your career. It was a great time for me as I was judged the best squadron leader of that year, and was asked to take over the role of 'Tac Ops', the chief observation officer and instructor.

I didn't accept it for two reasons. Firstly, I already had been pre-selected to go the new Army Personnel Centre (APC) in Glasgow, where I would be responsible for filling all staff vacancies requiring the rank of major. And secondly, Tania was pregnant again. Soon after returning from BATUS our daughter, Millie, was born in May 1999.

I loved the work at the APC and was getting super reports. However, Tania didn't move to Glasgow as there were not enough army quarters available. Uprooting her would have been miserable for her and therefore for me, so I took the option of renting a flat and commuting weekly from Yorkshire. In hindsight, that was probably the wrong thing to have done as there is little doubt that weekend-only couples grow more independent. Don't get me wrong; we were certainly not unhappy – on the contrary, it suited us both as I immersed myself in my work, returning each weekend to a lively household. But living apart, by its very definition, makes one more self-reliant.

After almost two years at Glasgow, I spent six months as second-in-command of the 1st Royal Tank Regiment that had unenthusiastically amalgamated with a squadron of the RAF Regiment to become the Joint Chemical, Biological, Radiological and Nuclear Regiment, then I moved to the MoD headquarters in London. Throughout this time, I continued to commute, allowing me to concentrate on my career during the week and Tania to enjoy the stability of living in Yorkshire.

I then landed one of my most rewarding jobs, commanding the Army Foundation College (AFC) in Harrogate. This amazing institution provides military training to junior soldiers aged between sixteen and seventeen. When I took over, I was responsible for the command of 1,600 teenagers and three hundred military staff without knowing any of my fellow officers. I often remarked that if I had been in charge of my own regiment – which I would have loved but there were undeniably better candidates than me – it would have been a far easier task. Commanding the Queen's Dragoon Guards is basically the same as commanding a squadron but on a larger scale and with more help. Not so at the AFC. Even more challenging was that I arrived in the middle of a media feeding frenzy after a highly publicised investigation into four recruits who had died between 1995 and 2002 in training at Deepcut. The initial inquest ruled that one of the deaths was suicide and gave an open verdict for the others. This was disputed by the trainee soldiers' families and the press, resulting in QC Nicholas Blake being commissioned to review the cases independently. He concluded that it was probable the deaths were self-inflicted, but criticised a number of aspects at Deepcut and the training centre which could be construed as having played a role in the suicides.

All this happened before I arrived, but I was now in the spotlight. To try and set the record straight, I told the press and members of the investigation teams that I had only recently taken on the job but welcomed the transparency. If I was not deemed to be doing the right thing, I wanted to know. We're the only army in the world that has sixteen-year-olds on the payroll and are regularly pilloried in the media for that. There are reasons why we do this, but I suggest you make up your own mind by watching a passing-out parade online. It's an extraordinary experience, watching parents dropping off their children at the beginning of the year and then returning twelve months later to find them confident, capable adults. Seven thousand people attend those parades and to see parents and relatives crying and ecstatically clapping is phenomenally moving.

I loved my time there. But as always, after two and a half years at the AFC I wanted to get some dust under my boots again. I volunteered to go to Afghanistan in the wake of the Second Gulf War and was embedded in the Office of Military Cooperation at the American headquarters in Kabul. My job was to facilitate recruiting and training new Afghan soldiers and advising their officers on how to run a modern army. I had the privilege of teaming up with General Sher Mohammad Karimi, chief of Afghanistan's army staff, who was very pro-British, having attended Sandhurst many years ago. He disliked flying, so we drove everywhere and as a result I visited many remote areas I barely knew existed. A particularly memorable trip was following the route of the infamous retreat from Kabul in 1842 during the First Anglo-Afghan War. It was one of our worst colonial disasters, in which more than 4,500 English soldiers and twelve thousand – mainly Indian – civilians accompanying them died either in fierce fighting or the brutal winter exposure. It culminated at the Battle of Gandamak, when twenty officers and forty-five soldiers of the 44th East Essex Regiment, armed with only twenty muskets and two shots per weapon, refused to surrender. They were all killed.

Amazing how history repeats itself, considering the Americans' equally disastrous withdrawal 179 years later in the summer of 2021. But at the time, we thought we were on the road to building a brave new modern country. The Americans were throwing so much money around that I was optimistic the Afghan army would prevail against the Taliban. In fact, during my six months there, there was only one car bomb – far removed from the chaos that exploded with a vengeance a decade later. I regularly went shopping in Kabul's bazaars with just a pistol tucked in my belt under my shirt.

From the worsening Afghan situation, although few suspected it at the time, I returned to Glasgow to run the branch responsible for the careers of all Royal Armoured Corps officers and soldiers. It was a great job and I chaired a number of boards assessing careers. As a result, many serving officers and soldiers thought I was more influential than I actually was. Take it from me: the process of career advancement in the Army is as fair as it can be.

I probably had ten years left in the military and, while I knew I would be lucky to be promoted to brigadier, it was not yet out of the question. However, I started to get itchy feet. I was now wearing a suit to work and felt more like a mandarin than anything else and decided I wanted one last foreign posting. I wanted to be a soldier again.

I applied for the position of deputy chief of staff of MONUC, a torturous French acronym for the UN peacekeeping mission in the Democratic Republic of the Congo. Although I suspected it was likely to be a routine job, at least it would mean I would be in Africa. The key stipulation was that the position had to be filled by a full colonel. Which I now was.

It turned out to be anything but routine.

12

Heart of Darkness

I didn't know much about the Democratic Republic of the Congo, although past experience has taught me always to be suspicious of countries that insert the word 'democratic' in their name.

What I did know was that it was vast – the eleventh-largest country in the world. It's also the fifth poorest, despite having untold reserves of diamonds, rare-earth minerals, cobalt, tin and copper. It's potentially richer in resources than all of western Europe.

Yet it's a borderline basket case. When I arrived, MONUC was the biggest peacekeeping mission ever undertaken by the UN, undertaken in response to what many call 'Africa's World War'. The flashpoint was the 1994 genocide in neighbouring Rwanda, resulting in the deadliest global conflict since the Second World War. Nine countries were sucked into the brutal vortex, resulting in an estimated 5.4 million deaths and twice that number of refugees.

Although the war ostensibly ended in 2003, hostilities certainly hadn't when I reported for duty seven years later. The country was reeling with several militant organisations and militias known as Mai-Mai, raping and pillaging at will.

My title was Deputy Chief of Staff (Forward), based in Goma, a shanty city on the Rwandan border. My small UN staff team of thirty was a thousand miles from headquarters in Kinshasa, but it could have been a million miles away, given the country's non-existent infrastructure. The only way we could get around efficiently was by helicopter.

The 'enemy' were the FDLR (Democratic Forces for the Liberation of Rwanda), a rebel group that fled their country after the genocide which their original leaders had largely instigated. However, today the FDLR is 40 per cent Congolese, not Rwandan, and has some popular support in the areas it has controlled for the last sixteen years. To finance themselves, the rebels ran unlicensed gold and tin mines and set up illegal roadblocks extorting money from motorists.

The UN's role was to support the authorities, but as the government forces were ill-disciplined, badly equipped and underpaid, with a human rights violations record as bad as the rebels, it was a messy situation.

An additional complication was that the UN brigades in the area were from India, Pakistan and Bangladesh, whose governments were mutually antagonistic. On behalf of my boss, General Babacar Gaye from Senegal, I was responsible for coordinating their operations and diplomacy was an absolute prerequisite. Fortunately, I got on well with the brigade commanders as the Indian subcontinent's armies have strong British links with a shared history and mutual respect.

Matters first came to a head after a massacre of villagers in a settlement called Hombo, which was in the Indian sphere of control, and the press hammered the UN for its perceived lack of effectiveness. However, there was not much the Indians could do within the terms of the UN's strict rules of engagement (or more correctly, non-engagement) and also the only road into Hombo was from the south, which was controlled by the Pakistanis.

When a second massacre in the same village occurred some months later, the UN was in real danger of being pilloried by all sides. Consequently, I received a call from Hiroute Guebre

Sellassie, head of the UN's Office of the North Kivu Area, demanding that the peacekeeping force 'did something'.

I called the brigade commanders and proposed that the Indians allow the Pakistanis to cross their 'border' to reach the village and at least investigate the perpetrators. Both said officially they couldn't do that – in fact, they weren't even supposed to be speaking to one another, given the sensitivity of the dispute over Kashmir. However, both agreed that the UN could 'order' the Indian brigade to let the Pakistanis through. In other words, all that was needed was a nod and a wink.

So I drafted an order from General Gaye giving instructions for the Pakistanis to send a road patrol into Indian-controlled Hombo to investigate the massacre. As soon as they were on their way, like a good staff officer I informed General Gaye what I had done on his behalf. In the British Army this is called 'mission command': officers are given the latitude to act within the commander's intentions. But General Gaye went ballistic, saying I had no idea of the 'complexity' of the situation. I have never received a bollocking like that from any superior officer, let alone a general. While I didn't accept that I'd made a mistake, I asked if he wanted to reverse the order. He said, 'No.' He was furious that I had gone above my station and issued an order resulting in sensitive troop movements, but I sensed he respected I had done the right thing. The main thing was that the UN was seen to be responding to a serious situation – an actual massacre of villagers – rather than hiding behind the walls of its fortified locations.

The highlights of the DRC tour of duty were meeting truly exceptional people. One outstanding example was Emmanuel de Merode, director of the Virunga National Park, a world-renowned habitat of the critically endangered mountain gorillas. Emmanuel is a scion of two of Belgium's most ancient and influential families, the Houses of Merode and Ligne, and is legally a prince, the title conferred upon his family by King Albert I in 1929. Obviously, he didn't use his blueblood credentials in the wilds of the Virunga Mountains and, believe me, they are wild. It's the oldest national park in Africa and he and his insanely brave rangers regularly have shootouts with heavily armed rebels, many of whom supplement their activities with poaching. In 2014, he was the target of an assassination attempt when gunmen pumped five AK-47 bullets into his chest and abdomen. Critically injured, he made it to the Goma hospital where doctors saved his life. That might have deterred a lesser man, but not Emmanuel. Today, he is still carrying on the good fight for the survival of these magnificent gentle giants and the environment in which they live.

I helped Emmanuel where I could, for example by ordering soldiers from the South African Engineer Battalion to prepare airstrips in the jungle from where his rangers could deploy. After all, I argued, the airstrips would also be useful to the UN when moving troops around by helicopter. He lived in a safari tent and I spent many enjoyable weekends in a clearing in the jungle, often watching movie classics such as *Battle of Britain*, *The Dam Busters* and *Casablanca* projected onto a white sheet as a screen.

Most remarkable of all of those I got to know was Gregory Alex, known to his legion of friends and admirers simply as Gromo. An American, he had headed the UN humanitarian assistance team in Kigali during the Rwandan genocide and saved hundreds of lives by delivering food and supplies to Tutsis hiding in safe houses. To do this, he had to bluff his way past checkpoints manned by machete-wielding Hutus, bartering for lives with little more than charm and chutzpah. His supreme courage, honesty and commitment to the people of Africa are unsurpassed. Sadly, he is no longer with us. He died in 2013.

Gromo ran DDR/RR (Disarmament, Demobilisation, Reintegration, Repatriation and Resettlement), a UN programme to disarm and repatriate Rwandan rebels still hiding in the DRC jungle. Less serious offenders guilty of genocide would be freed as long as they were genuinely remorseful, while the hardcore had to serve prison time. Gromo's team disarmed them and the Rwandan government assessed them.

Gromo had an office next to mine and we worked well together. When my six-month stint ended, I said to him that I would like to work with the DDR/RR and he replied they would like to have me. There were still thousands of rebels who needed to cross the line, and he said my military experience would be invaluable.

But the problem was that there were no British posts available, so we suggested to the UK government and the UN that I stay on as military liaison working with Gromo. They agreed and I took off my uniform, put on chinos and a checked shirt and carried on working for the UN as a civilian. It was a six-month contract. In the end, I stayed for twelve.

Our key method of communication was to set up radio stations as close to rebel and Mai-Mai militia camps as we could get, broadcasting lively music and messages and assuring rebels they would be treated well if they handed over their weapons. We had a number of these stations dotted around the area which I regularly visited, travelling either by myself or with an escort in more dangerous locations.

It worked well. In one case we heard about a high-profile intelligence officer in the FDLR who was keen to go home to his wife and kids. We picked him up in the bush and took him to Goma where we put him in a private prison – not to keep him in, but to keep irate members of the local community out. He was successfully repatriated to Rwanda.

On another occasion I 'reintegrated' a chap called Willie, the most senior Congolese member of ADF-Nalu, a militant Islamist group fighting to impose Sharia law in Uganda, but who had their base in the DRC. Willie phoned and said he wanted to hand himself over to 'the British colonel', as I was known. In those days, Britain was highly regarded in West and Central Africa, having successfully intervened in the Sierra Leone civil war a few years previously. We were keen on talking to Willie as we believed that ADF-Nalu was linked to Al-Shabaab in Somalia and Kenya. With the help of Miriam, a truly excellent UN field operative, I set up a meeting in a designated house. All we knew at that stage was that Willie was a nasty piece of work who had murdered either his father or brother. We didn't even know what he looked like, but I'd been told by a Senegalese officer who had been tracking him that he had no front teeth.

As I walked into the house unarmed, I noticed to my dismay that Willie did, in fact, have his incisors intact. I sat down and after a short while exchanging pleasantries said in French, 'Take out your teeth.' That would lead to one of two scenarios. Either he was not Willie or he had false teeth. No doubt surprised by my unexpected order, there was a moment's hesitation, but he knew I was not joking. He pulled them out and gave me a gap-toothed smile. We had our man.

Unfortunately, being Congolese, Willie didn't know much about the political aims of the Ugandan-based organisation he belonged to, so wasn't of much intel use. But at least we had got another bad bloke out of the bush.

I found myself in an equally bizarre situation when I flew into the jungle with Hiroute Guebre Sellassie, who had previously asked me to intervene in the Hombo massacres, to try and persuade the largest of the seventeen Mai-Mai groups to put down their weapons. Our helicopter landed on a football pitch three miles from the meeting place, so Hiroute had to stomp through thick mud and bush in high heels. An Ethiopian human rights lawyer, Hiroute was as tough as they come and had previously spent five years in an Addis Ababa jail for opposing the hardline Marxist dictator Mengistu Haile Mariam.

But if her wardrobe was out of place in the jungle, it was nothing compared to the rebels meeting us who were dressed, for some reason, in tutus. The Mai-Mai were infamous for their bizarre fashion sense, which was perhaps influenced by taking drugs in the belief that hallucinogens would turn bullets to water. But even so, to come across a muscular Mai-Mai with profoundly bloodshot eyes in a ballerina outfit is an image I won't forget.

However, the most intriguing incident of all was being offered the opportunity to exterminate the entire field leadership of the FDLR militants. It's something I still wonder about to this day.

I was doing some routine administrative stuff when Gromo called me to his office. 'There's a chap from France who wants to speak to you.' He handed me the phone.

'Is that Colonel Deacon?' The accent on the other end was distinctly African-French.

'Yes.'

'I would like you to help us with a problem with the FDLR.'

'How can we possibly help?' I asked.

The mystery voice continued, 'We are concerned that leaders in the field are not doing what they're told, and we want a political, not military, solution for Rwanda.'

'What's that got to do with me?'

'We can summon all FDLR leaders from the bush into one place through a radio call. Then we will tell you where they are and you can kill them all.' My silence confirmed my scepticism. 'We're serious. You can kill the lot and it will solve the Rwanda rebel problem.'

I told him I would get back to him.

This was intriguing but explosive stuff. Gromo and I decided to tell no one except a trusted senior British officer, and that I should travel to Paris and meet up with the mystery man to check his credibility.

I booked a room in the French Officers' Club, then selected a café on the corner of Rue Roy and Boulevard Haussmann with a decent vantage point and sent a message: 'I'll be sitting at a table in the corner wearing a green jersey and a red and yellow tie.' I figured that a green jersey might not stand out but was pretty sure there would be no one wearing the Royal Armoured Corps tie.

At 10 a.m. on the dot, a chap sat down opposite me. He was charming and no doubt deadly serious about his proposal.

He and the people he represented definitely – in my opinion – wanted to get rid of their commanders in the field and we were the perfect solution. One surgical strike by a helicopter gunship, of which MONUC had several, was all that was needed. I listened and drank my coffee, but made no promises for the simple reason that I couldn't.

Back in Goma we decided that, appealing as it was, the proposal was too farfetched to contemplate. For a start, the Indian brigade, who would be called upon to execute the helicopter strike, would rightly refuse to act on intelligence based on a dodgy conversation I'd had with a furtive man in Paris. Secondly, the UN contingents were paranoid about civilian collateral damage and feared reprisals.

My one shot at playing James Bond didn't come off.

After eighteen months in the cauldron of Africa, I returned to England and was awarded an OBE for the work I had done in disarming rebels. My small contribution had been recognised.

That was the good news.

The bad news, as the neurologist at the James Cook hospital succinctly put it, was that I had Parkinson's.

13

Parkinson's

To make the diagnosis crueller, I was about to start a fresh job as chief of staff, 2nd Division, based in Edinburgh. It was a job I wanted. But would the army still want me?

I rang the commander, Major-General David Shaw, the next day.

'I need to tell you something,' I said. 'I've got Parkinson's disease. I've just been diagnosed.'

He barely paused before answering. 'Sorry to hear that, but don't worry about it. Just carry on as normal.'

The relief was phenomenal. Most companies do their best to get rid of people with Parkinson's, believing that they can't do the job. The army is the other way around. It thinks of every reason it can to keep you – just as it does for people with multiple sclerosis and lost limbs. It recognised that there were many things I still could do, and for that I am forever grateful.

I started my new job in March 2011. 'HQ 2 Div', to use the vernacular, was based in Craigiehall, a seventeenth-century Scottish country house with beautiful grounds. The surrender of German forces in Norway was signed there in 1945. However, the house itself was only big enough for the officers' mess, so in the 1960s a prefab was erected, looking somewhat incongruous in the magnificent garden. We all worked there, keeping an eye on the four northern brigades in Preston, York, Belfast and Sterling. Despite its shabby exterior, the prefab was a happy headquarters, made all the more congenial by its rural surroundings. Tania and I were equally pleased with our own accommodation, a palatial stone house in the city centre and she landed an ideal job at Fettes College, one of the local public schools.

My Parkinson's was still in its early stages and the dopamine tablets worked well enough. I didn't notice much change, apart from getting a little slower and more tired. I also had the sense to realise it would be a good idea to talk to people in the same situation. Fortuitously, one of my closest friends is Georgina Matthews, whose sister Helen is now CEO of Cure Parkinson's. Helen's friend Tom Isaacs had contracted Parkinson's at just twenty-six and, to raise money for research, he walked the entire coastline of the UK. He completed the arduous 4,500-mile trek in a year, averaging sixteen miles a day, a remarkable achievement for anyone, let alone someone with Parkinson's. But equally astonishing was that he raised £350,000. Helen had assisted Tom on the coastal walk and with three other friends, they founded Cure Parkinson's in 2005.

I phoned Helen and was warmly accepted in the trust's fraternity. It's a fantastic organisation, and felt a bit like a club where they organise parties for members and raise loads of money. Every year the annual general meeting is in a fitting London venue and is great fun. It's the antithesis of a doom and gloom organisation, but they are laser-sharp in their focus. The name says it all – they want to find a cure. I have no doubt that they will achieve this noble goal, although I fear it will be too late for me. The answer is instead to work with what we've got and allow those yet to be diagnosed to benefit. Having said that, there are currently some promising trials, notably one with a drug called ambroxol which could result in something from which I could benefit.

But what could I do to help? I sort of knew the answer the moment I asked myself the question. I'd run marathons.

On the face of it, that seemed absurd. As a former rugby lock forward and more than six feet tall, I'm not built for long distance running which, in elite contests, favours small, wiry athletes – usually from Africa's Great Rift Valley. But non-elite marathon running is unlike almost any other sport in that the vast majority of contestants are only competing against themselves. Few care where so-and-so came, as the goal – apart from finishing – is to better your PB (personal best). I had previously completed a number of marathons and enjoyed the internal challenge. And that's what I decided to do for Cure Parkinson's.

I chose the Florence Marathon, a spectacular course weaving through the Renaissance city, mainly because it was six months away which gave me time to prepare. Despite Parkinson's, I was in reasonable shape physically, but not for a 26.2-mile marathon. So I laced up my trainers and went for a run.

A few weeks later I bumped into an old friend from my school days, Fiona Tanner. We ended up going out for dinner and during the course of the evening I mentioned I had Parkinson's. 'I'm running the Florence Marathon to raise funds to find a cure,' I said.

She didn't hesitate. 'I'm doing it with you.'

We started a training schedule, with me pounding the road in Scotland and her in London, comparing times and distances via text. Her support, even though virtual for most of the time, was a lifesaver and helped me emerge from the quicksand of despair that was in danger of consuming me.

Although not supremely fit, we both crossed the finishing line at the Piazza Santa Croce, a square overlooked by the Basilica of Santa Croce, Michelangelo's burial place. More importantly, we raised fifteen thousand pounds. Buoyed by the success, Fiona and I ran a second marathon in Barcelona, then a third in Budapest. All added to the Cure Parkinson's coffers.

Tania and I soon got used to living in Scotland. We both loved the freshness of the climate, the outdoors, walking the dogs, hiking, skiing and fishing. This was when I bought a Volkswagen campervan, the iconic brick-shaped 'surfer's van', which provided the mobility to turn the Scottish wilds into my backyard, opening the sliding door to some of the most exquisite scenery in the world. That freedom and solitude became a guardian angel, a soothing force of nature when my fear of the future bordered on dread.

I didn't know it then, but campervan exploring was later to become my focal point; the most challenging undertaking of my life. I think those days venturing deep into the Scottish backcountry in a beat-up Kombi campervan was a catalyst for my final odyssey.

I also loved shooting in Scotland as, having shot all my life, I now had the perfect wilderness on my doorstep. My favourite was stalking deer alone on the Amat estate in the Caledonian Forest where Tania's mother fortunately knew the owner. So it might come as a surprise to hear that I turned down an invitation to join the Queen at Balmoral.

OK, the invite didn't come from her majesty in person, of course. Instead, it was someone from the estate who recommended me. I had the credentials as I was a good shot, a cavalry colonel and, dare I say it, considered good company. Unless you're an ardent hunt saboteur or a dyed-in-the-wool republican, this is not an offer to turn down. But the shoot was scheduled for the next day, and with Parkinson's you need a little more time to get your head ready. And, of course, my self-confidence was low – one of the most pernicious side effects of the disease.

'I'm sorry, I have a meeting that I can't miss,' I said to the aide. 'Please pass on my thanks.'

Unsurprisingly, I was not asked again.

Slowly but surely, the disease squeezed its steel grip tighter and tighter. I found I was becoming increasingly exhausted. After lunch at work, I usually sneaked off for a nap. Even more embarrassingly, I'd fall asleep in meetings. I started stuttering more. The glib one-liners I was known for no longer tripped off my tongue. Although I wasn't the first person in the military to be diagnosed with Parkinson's, I was one of the few prepared to speak about it. I would rather people knew I had it than think I was a dopey git.

However, I had one more military job to do – and it turned out to be a really important one. I had thought the Congo mission would be my last career hurrah. I was wrong.

This one would be it.

I was appointed Colonel RAC, most easily described as head of the Royal Armoured Corps, an appointment held by a general when I first joined the army. This meant a move to Headquarters RAC, my old stamping ground at Bovington Camp, while Tania remained in Scotland to carry on teaching. She would commute south during the school holidays, while I dedicated my time to my work.

Colonel RAC is a job that can go either way. You either make it your legacy or sit back and wait out until your retirement. The choice is yours, and if you choose the latter, there are no recriminations, although it would mean your position was merely procedural and routine. For me, the choice was crucial. If I had taken the comfy option, it would effectively condemn me to sink meekly into Parkinson's oblivion.

I decided no. I would not go meekly. But it wasn't purely my resistance to Parkinson's that motivated me. It was a belief that the RAC had been unfairly shafted more regularly than any other branch of the armed forces of late and we had only ourselves to blame. There were several reasons for this, predominantly fostered by a growing belief that tanks were an anachronistic relic of the Cold War. Future wars, some were beginning to claim, would be along the lines of the insurgencies in Iraq and Afghanistan; hit-and-run guerrilla tactics or street fighting in areas with dense civilian populations. Consequently, appointments were increasingly held by infantry officers, leaving RAC officers in the margins and reducing chances of promotion. The Russian–Ukraine war has now indisputably demonstrated the need for a credible tank force, but at the time we were losing the argument before we had even made it.

Our problem, as far as I was concerned, was that the RAC consisted of nine seemingly different regiments that never spoke with one voice to justify our role. Cavalry regiments are among the oldest in the British Army and extremely proud ones. We urgently needed to coordinate the debate about our immense value to the British Army and provide strategic thinking on how the RAC could best provide an armoured capability to the UK's defence. In short, we needed not only to defend our case, but to trumpet it. That became my mission.

I succeeded. I was awarded a CBE for my efforts. However, I unreservedly dedicate that award to my staff. I would never have achieved the results I wanted without 'mission command', the same tactic I had used with the Indian and Pakistani brigades in the DRC. Except this time, it was reversed; I was now relying on trusted officers on the ground to use their initiative. I gave them a task and the resources they needed, but never micromanaged them.

Among my team's many achievements was forming a RAC Council, a powerful group of brigadiers that coordinated the development of the corps and its staff. It briefed very senior officers with an agreed line and they began to make things happen in the top echelons of the army.

I often joked the award indicated that the Queen had forgiven my Balmoral stalking snub in the infinitely unlikely event that she even knew about it. But I cannot over-emphasise how much my time as Colonel RAC meant to me. I left the army with the satisfaction of a job well done. Without that to focus my efforts, and with Parkinson's in fast progression, I might well have retired in a stupor, overcome and wallowing in self-pity.

I avoided that fate because the British Army is a fabulous employer. It never once wavered and kept confidence in me even though they were aware the disease was stalking me like a horseman of the apocalypse. My gratitude for that and for the senior officers surrounding me in my time of need is incalculable.

But it was now time to go.

On my bad days, I couldn't get off the floor, I was so depressed and debilitated. I had begun to shuffle, wearing out shoes at an alarming rate, while the pills made my legs swell so much that I couldn't get my boots on under my mess kit trousers. At formal functions I rarely ate food as I couldn't cut it into bite-size chunks – and there was no way I was going to ask anyone, particularly perfect strangers, to do that for me.

It was time to follow another dream and, as it had before, Africa beckoned.

While the past few years as Colonel RAC had been my last hurrah, this – my last great adventure – would be an odyssey.

14

Start of the Odyssey

To call a trip through Africa an odyssey may sound a little grandiose, particularly as at this stage my goals weren't clearly defined. To fulfil a childhood dream, combined with a love of wild camping, vast open spaces and a new VW campervan campervan, simply seemed to be as good an idea as any at the time.

But even so, I reckon for someone who'd lived with Parkinson's for a decade, this was more than just a trip. It was indeed, for me anyway, an odyssey.

When I say the campervan was 'new', it was only in the sense that I had recently acquired it. In reality, it was five years old and had thirty thousand miles on the clock. My old Kombi, which provided such pleasure roaming the Scottish wilderness, had given up the ghost and, feeling lost without it, I had found the lovely silver-grey Volkswagen with a legendary two-litre TDI engine and a pop-top roof. Like my previous van, it was four-wheel drive, allowing me to go off the beaten track. It was exactly what I wanted and certainly up for the job I had in mind. From then on, the van affectionately became known as 'the wagon'.

But first, as I was about to leave the Army, I had to attend a week-long senior officers' resettlement course. The Army invests in you, whether you like it or not, and this course was specifically designed to equip departing officers with job skills that would be useful in civilian life. It was excellent, teaching us how to run our own websites, how to network in a business environment, choosing suitable roles and how to manage finances. We could select whatever course we wanted, from bricklaying to accountancy, and many chose to go to business schools. Equally useful was that each participant had a personal tutor to advise and coach them for job interviews.

My tutor ended up in a bit of a quandary when she asked what I wanted to do.

'Well... I'm not sure I'm meant to be here,' I replied. 'I don't actually want a job.'

She looked at me askance. No doubt I was the first interviewee to have said that to her. I explained that I had Parkinson's and would be able to live on my Army pension if I reduced my costs. Also, my wife was still working, our children had left home and I had no grand aspirations for a big house, flashy cars or extravagant holidays. 'But I have a plan,' I said.

'What's that?'

'To drive to Sierra Leone and beyond.' I didn't expand, as I still wasn't sure what 'beyond' would be at the time.

She mulled that over. 'OK, what you should do is give yourself a solid reason for doing the journey,' she said. 'Instead of just disappearing and travelling willy-nilly, you ought to have a sense of purpose. Make the trip have meaning, not just something to do for the sake of doing it.'

That sounded simple, but was actually profound advice. She was a highly astute tutor and well aware that people who say they don't want a job often run the risk of sinking into lethargy. Particularly if they are suffering from a debilitating, incurable disease. So, although the resettlement course had not specifically prepared me for a new job – obviously, because I didn't want one – the tutor had in effect helped me resolve what to do next with my life. Instead of just wandering off, I should give my plan a more tangible focus. Make it a life's goal. In other words, an odyssey.

As it happened, I did have a reason to make the journey – although pretty vague at the time. I did not envisage my trip purely as a ramble through deserts and jungles with starlit nights in the bush. I wanted to raise awareness of Parkinson's on my travels.

This too was not just a lightbulb moment. I was well aware that people afflicted with Parkinson's in Africa have an even more challenging time than those in other parts of the world. I was particularly moved by work being done by Parkinson's Africa, a charity founded by an exceptionally courageous Nigerian woman, Omotola Thomas, who had been diagnosed with the disease when only thirty-five. Omotola is a tireless campaigner for the estimated 2.2 million sufferers in Africa where effective medicine is not affordable – or even accessible – in many areas. This is further exacerbated, says Omotola, by ignorance of the disease resulting in sufferers often being stigmatised.

Despite everything, I was one of the lucky ones with Parkinson's. My treatment is the best available in the world and I can barely imagine how any sufferer copes without the help that I have. Aside from the devastating physical symptoms of Parkinson's, without dopamine enhancer medication the chronic depression, strength-sapping fatigue and crippling anxiety attacks can be totally overwhelming. And millions of people face that dire situation every day of their lives.

Maybe in some small way I could help. Perhaps, by making more people aware, I could shine a ray of light on what living with Parkinson's was actually like. So I went to Helen Matthews, CEO of Cure Parkinson's and told her what I planned to do. I was not proposing a straightforward fundraising mission – in fact, that was not even the key aim. As far as that was concerned, I had already tapped everyone I knew when raising money by running marathons. Instead, by focusing on awareness I would attempt to show that having Parkinson's does not mean giving up on life. Sufferers can still achieve goals and do things they want to if they have help. Help that many in Africa just don't have. The message was simple – don't be defeated – and I hoped it would be powerful.

Helen was supportive as always, appointing me a Cure Parkinson's ambassador while the charity enthusiastically endorsed the trip.

Four weeks later, the African Odyssey started, as I drove my van – the wagon – decked out with Cure Parkinson's logos through the front gates of Sherborne School. I had been boarding with my good friend Andrew Spink while I got everything ready and just before leaving, his wife Sue said we ought to get some publicity. She's a marketing expert and arranged for Helen Matthews to be on hand. As both Andrew and I were Sherborne old boys, the school's spectacular driveway was designated the official departure point, as it would provide a great photo opportunity.

In retrospect, that was a good idea; when the photo appeared in the local newspaper a couple of weeks later, it sparked considerable media interest, and I was even interviewed by CNN. But at the time I didn't want publicity. I just wanted to be on the road, yearning for the simplicity which campervan travel affords. In fact, my only social media was a page on Polarsteps, a website used mainly by travellers or adventurers embarking on unusual voyages. I guess mine was as strange as any other.

For a start, I had limited use of my hands, poor spatial awareness and sometimes appeared drunk to those who did not understand Parkinson's. I also would be navigating by GPS in areas where roads weren't marked or where satellite reception was not guaranteed, sleeping in the bush often hundreds of miles from any settlement. I suppose some might think that crazy.

James Moberly, one of my best friends from Durham University and Sandhurst, joined me for the first few days. I picked him up at Camberley before heading for Newhaven to catch the ferry to Dieppe. Even though the trip was about Africa, I still had to drive south through Europe to get there and I wasn't about to skimp on that. Dieppe was high on my to-do list, particularly the beaches where the famous Second World War raid led by the Canadians in 1942 took place. This was two years before D-Day and it was a disaster, with the landing craft running into a German convoy that opened fire, alerting the coastal defences. About two thousand soldiers died, a thousand of whom were from Canada. As a cavalry officer I could empathise with the crewmen of the Churchill tanks that were bogged down on the shingle beaches – two sank in deep water – while all hell broke loose. All tank crews that landed on the beach were either killed or captured.

Our visit was sombre and in my Parkinson's-withered state, it was an apt time to be reminded of the ultimate sacrifice so many men and women made during both wars. As ex-military men, James and I saluted them on the beach with absolute respect.

We didn't speak much about my Parkinson's while we were together. We didn't need to: it is what it is. I simply knew that James would always be there for me and such things do not need to be said. He came along with me as a good mate, not to commiserate, but to enjoy life. That we did in abundance with good food, wine and companionship.

I am truly blessed with such friends. Another was Andrew Hartley, leader of the university's Turkana expedition many years earlier, whom I picked up in Paris a day after dropping James off. I always joke that Andrew turns up like a bent penny and it is true. He is a breath of fresh air no matter where or when we meet up, be it Kenya or France, Istanbul or the Congo. He has a knack of getting into trouble and an equally uncanny knack of getting out of it. A more loyal fellow you could not meet.

I spent three or four days with Andrew and his wife Sylvie, drinking wine and reliving past adventures, some of which are unsuitable to repeat in polite company. In fact, many of the stories we do repeat have grown more and more inaccurate over time, yet we still find them hilarious – even if no one else does.

I dropped Andrew off at Chenonceaux and headed south towards Limoges, where I first encountered what would become a recurring theme of the journey: the incredible kindness of strangers. Before leaving the UK, I mentioned to a friend, Chris Forrest, that I would be in France and his mother – who I had never met before – unhesitatingly handed me the keys to her house in Limoges, saying I could stay for as long as I liked. 'Even if you just knock on the door, the neighbours will let you in,' she said. That was exactly what happened and I rested there for a couple of days in the beautiful countryside, rearranging stowage in the wagon and drinking the local hooch with neighbours Francoise and Xavier before pointing the wagon south towards Carcassonne, a mediaeval city not far from the Mediterranean. I like travelling at night when the roads are quieter and just before arriving at the walled city I turned down a muddy track to camp in the woods. A few minutes later I reversed into a hidden ditch with an ominous metallic clunk.

Dammit! The diff's gone, was my immediate thought: the 'differential gears' constantly adjust the power to the wheels.

But as no dashboard warning light flashed and the vehicle kept going, I couldn't be sure. I spent the night parked in the woods and, after a hasty breakfast, drove to the nearest VW garage. The mechanic did an electronic diagnostics check, but couldn't find anything wrong with the diff. One gave me a thumbs up and simply said, '*Bien.*' It was good to go.

I was not convinced. But who was I to argue with French mechanics and a fancy computer?

That night I drove gingerly up into the Pyrenees mountains and into Andorra, sandwiched between France and Spain. It was not on my original itinerary, but I'd never been there before so decided on an impromptu visit. It's a good thing that I did.

In fact, it would probably have been catastrophic if I hadn't.

15

Jimmy and Mohammed

It was 2 a.m. and pitch-dark when I arrived in the principality and I decided to camp in the snow on one of the passes through the ring of mountains surrounding the capital, Andorra la Vella.

I love wild camping and avoid campsites as much as possible, preferring solitude to screaming kids and shops that sell soap powder and flip-flops. Whenever I can, I hide in the woods or fields and that's why I bought the 4x4 van – to go off the beaten track. I would either pop the roof and sleep upstairs or rearrange the stowage and make up a simple bed. As it's extremely difficult for me to get in a sleeping bag or even cope with normal bedding, I usually sleep in a soft overcoat and fleecy, zip-up trousers. In some of the dodgier places, I would just crank the seat back and catnap until sunrise.

Still worried about the rear differential, I drove to Andorra's Volkswagen dealership as it opened, forgetting it was Saturday. Their sales team told me to come back on Monday so, with nothing to do but wait, I checked into the city's only campsite. As it was early winter, there was only one other camper and his wife, in a large converted Mercedes charabanc. As the vehicle had a British number plate, I went over to introduce myself.

His name was Jimmy Thomas and he turned out to be a real character. Originally from Lancaster, he now lived in Majorca and, as his summer job was providing jet skis for Mediterranean luxury yachts, he was good with engines. He was also an avid biker and in winter would load up his motorhome with motorbikes to ride the challenging Pyrenees mountain passes. That's what I love about travelling – I would never have met someone like Jimmy in everyday life.

In the course of our conversation, I mentioned I had a problem with the van and without hesitation he said, 'Let's have a look at it.' He crawled under the vehicle, took off the bash plate – a solid aluminium sheet that provides an underbody shield against rocks – then poked his head out from below. 'There's an oil leak here. Not good.' I nodded. He had confirmed my suspicions. 'Tell you what, I know someone who can help. My mate Mohammed.' He pulled out his mobile phone and after a brief conversation in Spanish, he turned to me. 'Mohammed used to own a garage close to the campsite, but there's not enough business to keep him going. He's off home to Morocco in a couple of weeks. We caught him just in time.'

Mohammed arrived the next day. Wearing jeans and a black leather jacket, he was tall and gangly and smiled a lot. I liked him instantly, communicating in French, a second language for both of us. We had barely shaken hands before he and Jimmy were under the van. 'Not good,' Mohammed said, echoing Jimmy's verdict.

Fortunately, Mohammed knew a place where we could get diagonally opposite wheels off the ground and check the diff by spinning them. In less than thirty minutes he'd found the problem that had stumped the computer and factory-trained French mechanics. 'The diff's broken,' was the bad news. Just as I had thought.

But where to get a new one? England? That would take several weeks. Volkswagen make regular improvements to their California campervans so it was really important to get the right year for the vehicle and the part. While I was wondering what to do next, Jimmy was already one step ahead and on the phone.

I think he phoned every dealership in Europe. Eventually, after two days, he struck gold. An outlet in Holland had the right model and they would ship it within a week.

That prolonged my stay in Andorra by seven days. To pass the time, Jimmy and I drank lots of beer, ate fish and chips and went for walks in the mountains. He'd seen the Cure Parkinson's logo on the van and I told him what my trip to Africa was all about. He'd heard enough about the disease to know that what I was attempting was going to be a challenge and was really supportive. As was Mohammed, but in a different way.

One day he handed me a marijuana joint. It was the size and thickness of a Cuban cigar. 'Morocco's finest,' he said. 'Good for Parkinson's.'

That might sound crazy but there is indeed a school of thought that believes weed is beneficial for Parkinson's sufferers. However, I hadn't smoked the stuff for more than thirty-five years – it's not something colonels in the British Army do. I put it to one side until, that night while reading a book in the van, I noticed Mohammed's joint 'staring' at me. I'm not convinced about the medicinal benefits, but thought, Why not? and lit up. Disappointingly, it had no effect. I smoked it harder. Still no effect. I eventually smoked the entire reefer in one session.

Then without warning, waves of woozy nausea engulfed me. I swivelled my chair around and opened the sliding door, sat on the floor of the van and dangled my feet outside. It was just in time as moments later I was violently ill, aiming for the ground but spewing mostly onto my shoes and trousers. Icy air blasted down from the snow-peaked mountains, but I was so stoned I couldn't move out of the cold. Head spinning crazily, all I could think of was that I was about to die of exposure and the screaming headline story in the British tabloids would be 'Retired colonel found dead in snow drift after smoking dope in mountains'.

I knew I had to get my medication quickly. The pills were in the front of the van and somehow I managed to ease out of the back. Clinging to whatever I could – handles, mirrors, windscreen wipers – I edged towards the passenger's door. It must have taken me half an hour to get there, then pop open the blister pack of pills with my terrible coordination and swallow a handful. Gradually, I started to recover and realised that I had to clean myself up. I stumbled to the shower block and jumped under the steaming hot water fully clothed, as I needed to wash the mess off them as well. Once scrubbed, I put on a thin Kenyan kikoi – a kind of sarong – and walked back to the van with my wet clothes over my arm. With the heater blasting, the van was soon toasty again.

The next day I bumped into Jimmy. 'Have a good evening, mate?

'Absolutely fine, thank you.' I was in no mood to tell the truth.

Not long afterwards, Mohammed arrived. Making a smoking sign with his hands, he asked, 'Did you enjoy it?'

'Excellent, *mon ami*. Thank you very much.'

When the differential arrived, we had another problem. Andorra is not part of the European Union so we couldn't bring it across the border. There was import tax and a mountain of paperwork to complete, which Mohammed sorted out for me. Then he and Jimmy fitted the part and an hour or so later the wagon was good to go. Mohammed charged a pittance for the job, and even that he did reluctantly. Nothing was said, but I think both he and Jimmy respected what I was trying to do in my debilitated condition and this was their way of showing it.

Before leaving Andorra, Mohammed drove me to shops in the city belonging to friends and relatives, saying I needed to stock up for the next leg of the trip. I soon realised this was no ordinary shopping trip when he started pulling stuff off the shelves.

'You'll need some of these,' he said, grabbing an armful of courgettes. 'Do you like avocados?' he asked as we passed another shelf, stuffing them into another bag without waiting for an answer. The same with pineapples and nuts. I certainly wouldn't starve on my way down.

Neither he nor his friends would take any money. I was speechless; I had never encountered such extraordinary generosity – and from complete strangers.

Knowing that Morocco was going to be my first stop in Africa, Mohammed urged me to meet him in two weeks' time at his home in Larache, a coastal city in the north-west of the country. I wasn't sure if he meant it, but vowed that I would make the attempt after all he had done for me. Besides, I really liked him.

I crossed into Spain, where I'd originally planned to spend some time visiting the battlefields of the Peninsular War of the early nineteenth century. But after my enforced downtime in Andorra I now had to hurry and drove through the country in a day as I was scheduled to meet two expats in Portugal. One was Christina Hippisley, who'd very kindly brought over the spare van keys that I'd left behind in England.

The other was the mother of Charlotte 'Charlie' le Poidevin. I'd met Charlie in Bovington and we had become friends after she kept rescuing my wayward labrador, who had an annoying habit of wandering away from home. She was young and strong and I think looked on me as a dishevelled father figure who, suffering from a debilitating disease, needed help. Which I did, as I had to move all the stuff from my army house into storage. This included spare tyres, toolboxes, cupboards, a washing machine and fridge-freezer, so was not a one-man job – certainly not a one-man-with-Parkinson's job. I simply couldn't have done it without her and when she heard that I would be travelling through Portugal, she said I should visit her mum, Sue, who emigrated some time ago and unreservedly welcomed a complete stranger simply because I vaguely knew her daughter in another country.

I could only stay for a short while and Sue helped me complete some minor tasks such as blacking out the van's rear windows to give some privacy on my travels. That evening, stuck for something to keep us occupied, I encouraged her to watch *Love and Other Drugs*, the best Hollywood movie about Parkinson's ever made. It's lighthearted and jolly but doesn't gloss over the bad bits. The only thing I forgot to mention, having seen it so often, is that it's very much adult humour. I seem to remember Charlie's mum saying, 'That's a bit unusual,' as actress Anne Hathaway removed her clothing yet again!

Next stop was Gibraltar, my final European destination. It's a soldier's place: a heavily fortified military garrison and strategic naval base that Britain acquired from Spain in 1713. Although the territory comprises only 2.6 square miles, it controls the entrance to the Mediterranean.

As I crossed the border and asked directions to the campsite, a customs official said it was illegal to camp anywhere on the tiny peninsula. But, she said, I can go to the carpark at the South Artillery Battery where 'some people spend a lot of time'.

'But don't camp,' she said with a slight smile.

I also foolishly tried to draw some cash. Changing money was to become a regular challenge at most border posts and while I had dollars and euros, I believed that the good old pound sterling would also be useful and went to an ATM. My Lloyds debit card was to take a fair old hammering over the next months and rarely let me down. But it certainly did on this occasion – the machine whirred into action and spewed out Gibraltar pounds, which are worthless anywhere else in the world. You can't even use them in the UK. So, armed with wedges of monopoly money, I went to Morrisons supermarket and bought as much non-perishable food as I could carry.

Loaded with peanut butter, Marmite, sardines, crackers and goodness knows what else, I left Gibraltar for Algeciras and caught the car ferry to Africa.

The odyssey was about to begin in earnest.

16

Morocco

This time around, my first step in Africa was on what is technically Spanish soil.

It's a tiny peninsula called Ceuta, an autonomous Spanish port that juts into Morocco. In other words, a mirror image of Gibraltar on the other side of the Mediterranean. Unsurprisingly, Morocco wants Ceuta and the other autonomous city on the African mainland, Melilla, back – just as Spain wants Gibraltar. This perhaps makes Spain uncomfortably open to the charge of hypocrisy: it has occupied its two enclaves for as long as Britain has had Gibraltar and has no intention of giving them up. That doesn't stop the Spaniards from claiming Gibraltar as theirs – despite the people actually living there voting to remain with Britain by a whopping 98.97 per cent in the 2002 sovereignty referendum.

But duplicitous politics were far from my mind as I drove off the ferry. Instead, I followed a handwritten sign pointing towards the border post and found myself in a car park with hundreds of other vehicles. The park's holding area was bigger than central Ceuta itself, which reminded me of Gibraltar but far dirtier.

There I waited. And waited. Every now and again there would be some movement for no apparent reason and we would shift forward a few yards, then continue waiting. Eight hours later, well after midnight, I reached the actual border and handed over my passport to stony-faced officials. It reminded me of the movie *Midnight Express*; after waiting another half-hour to get an array of forms stamped, I was finally in Morocco.

It was now about 3 a.m. but I was wide awake – one symptom of Parkinson's is an inability to sleep well – and I started heading south. That was the plan. But like all best-laid plans, it was soon thwarted. This time by a piece of string. Well, not by the string itself, but rather the policeman sitting on a stool who was holding one end of it. The other end was attached to a crash barrier.

This was my first of many encounters with a Moroccan vehicle checkpoint and at first I thought it was a scam to extort money. But Morocco is not a poor country. It ranks above India in GDP per household. So why a string roadblock? I braked and wound down my window. The policeman stood and smiled in the semi-darkness. His face was pleasant and his pistol remained holstered, which is always a good sign.

'Documentation,' he asked, holding out a hand.

I was prepared for this and had been advised beforehand to get a *fiche* – an A4-sized document containing all one's personal and vehicle particulars which saves you having to do so verbally at each checkpoint. And believe me, there're a lot of them. I had about forty *fiche* printed and used them all. But I wasn't prepared for the next question.

'Insurance?'

He had me there. As it's impossible to buy vehicle insurance for Africa within Europe, I'd planned to get the necessary documentation at Ceuta. I couldn't find anywhere to do that once across the border, so decided to buy insurance when I arrived at the next town – hopefully without crashing into anything. I explained that to the policeman and he instructed me to go back to Tangiers, the main Moroccan ferry port, and get insured there. He gave vague directions where to find a broker at the docks.

Tangiers was about fifty miles in the opposite direction. I was tired and frustrated after the long wait at the Ceuta border and it had been some time since I had taken my medication. And now – before I had even begun – I was required to go back to square one. That's one of the main problems with Parkinson's; stress exacerbates the symptoms and even minor issues can grow out of all proportion. I needed to calm down. I pointed to a layby on the side of the checkpoint. 'May I rest there for a while?'

The policeman smiled. 'Of course.'

Consequently, my first night in Africa was spent at a checkpoint. Something I would do many more times.

I arrived in Tangiers the next day and followed the policeman's directions in a quest to find an insurance broker. Despite poor signage, I did – but it was hardly Lloyd's of London. In fact, the man I was looking for was sitting in a small shed, on a stool behind a table that would have looked more at home in the nearby fish market. I handed over some cash as he scribbled something in Arabic onto a strip of coloured paper, which he then tore from a sheet and gave to me. My van was now legal in Morocco and Western Sahara for the next three months. Or that's what I hoped he said.

I had ten days to kill before my scheduled meeting with Mohammed the mechanic from Andorra and I headed down the Atlantic coast for a campsite at Kénitra on the banks of the Sebou River that flows majestically down the Atlas Mountains. It was magnificent, a beautiful resort with big sandy beaches where I could sip a cold beer while watching colourful wooden fishing boats bob in the estuary as the sun set. It was an instant antidote to any Parkinson's-induced agitation.

After two days, I headed inland towards Chefchaouen, the famed so-called 'Blue City' as for some reason most of it is painted blue. People rave about it, but what struck me more than the thousands of blueish buildings were the hordes of foreign backpackers hanging around, drinking and smoking.

I was underwhelmed, but it was late, I needed somewhere to stay and drove around searching for a campsite. I saw a sign advertising exactly that, but once I had paid a paltry sum to a distinctly unwelcoming man with few teeth, I noticed it was more of a scrapyard than anything else.

After parking the wagon, I noticed a Land Rover that looked less decrepit than the other vehicles and walked over, thinking it belonged to overlanders – people travelling all the way down the continent to South Africa. It wasn't a group of intrepid travellers at all. In fact, the engine was in pieces and inside the vehicle sat a couple of unsavoury-looking locals smoking dope. They stared at me sullenly. At that point I realised that not only was I the sole camper in the 'camp', I was the only person not stoned.

Feeling distinctly uneasy, I manoeuvred the wagon to point towards the gate for a quick getaway if necessary and mentally devised an escape plan. It was pretty basic: I would sleep in the top, fully clothed, in order to quickly slide down into the driver's seat, fire up the wagon (even though the buzzers and alarms would be blaring to remind me to shut the roof), thump it into gear and crash through the barrier to make my getaway. If I ended up trailing power cables and the awning or roof got damaged it would be a small price to pay for my safety. I carried no weapons, believing that if I needed them I would be in deeper trouble than they would be useful for, but had two pepper-spray aerosols stashed in the pockets of each front door. The last straw would be to bore any assailant to death by moving absurdly slowly – pretty easy with Parkinson's – and charm.

Unsurprisingly, I didn't have a wink of sleep that night and left before sunrise, expecting the roads to be empty.

Not bloody likely! Almost immediately, I found myself behind a slow-moving flatbed truck with a bulldozer on the back that obstructed my view. To overtake it with my right-hand drive van, I had to pull far over the road to see ahead. At that precise moment another ill-lit lorry came hurtling around a corner. It happened so fast that there was nothing I could do except try squeezing between the two juggernauts. That I didn't lose both wing mirrors, let alone the wagon, was a miracle. Surprised I was still in one piece, I pulled in at the next safe place to calm down.

Next stop was the Roman ruins of Volubilis and the imperial city of Meknes. As it was winter, there were no tourists and I had the UNESCO World Heritage Site to myself. Exceptionally well-preserved with many fine mosaics, the city was a sobering reminder that the Romans were there long before the rest of us and that time is fleeting. A sombre reflection for someone in my condition and, indeed, I was finding this trip was increasingly becoming the odyssey I had envisaged. This was further shown when I stumbled upon a travelling *souk* near the ruins frequented solely by locals, where I bought a woollen Berber cloak, which meant infinitely more to me than the tourist-riddled Blue City.

Although I'd had WhatsApp communication with Mohammed, I still wasn't sure if we'd meet up in Larache but was determined to keep my end of the bargain and headed for the coast. As I approached the city outskirts, I was initially unimpressed; it looked almost abandoned, with dozens of huge unoccupied apartment blocks. But Larache's *medina* – which in North African cities refers to a historic quarter with winding streets and narrow alleyways – was charming. This was the Morocco I had envisaged.

While looking for a campsite, I noticed an overland truck in a car park in the middle of town and decided to camp there for the night. I had just settled down for a meal of dates and pasta – my staple diet – when I had a visitor.

'Why are you here?' It was the car park guard. He was a bit officious and I thought he was going to tell me to leave or demand money. However, he was merely interested to know what I was doing and had come over for a chat. That was the last thing I wanted as he had caught me at a low point. My medication was wearing off and I was becoming a gibbering wreck. Whenever that happens, I need time to myself. But he refused to be fobbed off, so eventually I said, 'I'm here to meet a friend.'

'What's his name?'

Finding it hard to concentrate and not wishing to explain myself, I just shook my head, trying to wave him away.

'What's his name?' the car guard repeated with more authority.

'Umm... Mohammed.' Even to me that sounded lame. Mohammed was Morocco's most common name. In fact, not just in Morocco, but in the entire Islamic world.

'Let's go and look for him,' said the guard.

My eyes rolled. I desperately needed a lie-down. 'No. He's only coming tomorrow.'

'We go now.'

He could see the exasperation on my face and perhaps thought it was because we were both speaking in French. He then whistled over another chap who spoke some English. To my growing agitation, I had to repeat my story about meeting Mohammed who was only coming tomorrow.

'We find him now. Follow me.' The interpreter tugged at my sleeve.

It seemed simpler to go with the flow rather than continue arguing, so I followed him and the guard up some stone stairs leading to the *medina*. Washing hung between paint-flaked buildings and at the top of the stairs sat an old man smoking a hookah pipe with a small cup of mud-coloured coffee balanced on a table in front of him. He was wearing jeans, a black puffer jacket and a blue beanie and looked about a hundred, although he was probably in his seventies. His eyes sparkled in a weathered face etched with humour and a lifetime of experience.

'Is this your Mohammed?' the car park guard asked.

If it was, Mohammed the mechanic had aged dramatically in the trip over from Andorra. 'No,' I said. This was becoming painful.

'I am Mohammed,' said the old man.

'But not the Mohammed I know,' I replied.

'No, I am his uncle. He and I are meeting you tomorrow.'

'Mohammed from Andorra? He's your nephew?' I asked incredulously.

He nodded. I sucked in a lungful of air. The coincidence was simply staggering.

Uncle Mohammed then invited me into his nearby shop which at first glance seemed to be selling paintings and carpets. But, incongruously, stashed in among some *kasbah* clutter, was a wealth of old rock'n'roll posters and a fabulous collection of vinyl records. The old man had been a roadie for Jimi Hendrix and various other bands who had played at festivals in Marrakesh during the 1960s. The city had been an iconic stopover on the hashish hippie trail, immortalised by Crosby, Stills & Nash in their hit song 'Marrakesh Express'. Sensing my amazement, he showed me newspaper cuttings which told stories of wild nights for both rock stars and fans. Mohammed said that whenever big bands such as Pink Floyd had come to Morocco, he was their go-to man, fixing accommodation and meals and generally making sure they were well catered for. Judging by the large joint the old man was smoking, I guess that also meant a supply of wacky baccy. I spent a hugely entertaining couple of hours talking to him – or rather listening, as he was doing all the talking.

Next morning, I rang Mohammed the mechanic, who said he had just arrived and would meet me at his rock'n'roll uncle's shop. After some hugging and back-slapping, we walked to a café for coffee with Uncle Mohammed, still as lively and entertaining as he had been the day before. Nephew Mohammed then showed me his city, much of which I had seen when I arrived, but it was far more interesting to view it through a local's eyes. After that, we went to his parents' house for lunch.

Mohammed's father was a retired truck driver and in fifty years on the road had not had a single accident. His mother greeted me warmly, then retired to the kitchen to cook. Their hospitality was immaculate. While waiting for lunch, Mohammed's father noticed I looked tired and, knowing about my disease, immediately made up a bed complete with sheets in the sitting room where I slept for an hour to regain my strength. When lunch was served – a delicious dish of fish and vegetables – he put the food on a fork for me so that I didn't have to chase it around the plate. He didn't try and feed me but he just unobtrusively and politely made sure what I needed was on my fork. Neither parent spoke French, so Mohammed had to translate everything, which made conversation a bit stilted. But he was so proud of his parents and his English friend – stricken as I was – that it was a truly memorable meal.

Mohammed then arranged for us to spend the night at a friend's beach house about forty-five minutes north of Larache. We stopped en route at a roadside café which, he said, served the best burgers not only in Morocco, but in the world. Looking at the garish neon lights and plastic chairs and tables, I was far from convinced. Also, to dine out on humble burgers in an exotic country such as Morocco would surely be a serious culinary anti-climax.

I watched with interest as the chef sliced a giant steak off a hunk of beef hanging from a hook on a rafter, mincing it with a little fat in an ancient hand-grinder, then throwing in some North African herbs and spices. After sizzling the patty on a cast-iron skillet, he served it in a freshly baked bread roll with chips and vegetables. It was a virtuoso performance – and one of the most delicious meals I've had. Just as Mohammed promised.

If I thought being served a meal worthy of five Michelin stars in a Moroccan greasy spoon was strange, the rest of the evening was even more bizarre. When we arrived at Mohammed's friend's – still uncompleted – house at the top of a lane overlooking the sea, he pulled out a carrier bag full of cannabis. I suspected he wanted to give me some as I hadn't yet had the heart to tell him that the first spliff in Andorra nearly killed me. But this was a batch of weed we first needed to process as the stalks and seeds were still attached.

There was a security guard outside, so Mohammed also invited him in to help. I couldn't help reflecting on the *Monty Python*-esque situation – a former British cavalry colonel suffering from Parkinson's with a Moroccan mechanic half his age and a penniless security guard all amiably processing dope together. I wasn't much help as not only had I never done this before, but my lack of motor skills made it extremely difficult to separate a single leaf from a stalk.

All I knew was that the next day sanity would prevail. I would soon be meeting my wife and daughter at Marrakesh to spend Christmas in the Atlas Mountains.

But first I needed to do a quick detour to the capital city, Rabat.

17

Snow, Sand and Surf

Before setting off to Africa, I had decided not to call on British embassies as I didn't expect support. However, as an ex-army man, I did plan to pay my respects to various defence attachés, as we would have an instant connection with our shared military credentials. Also, my experiences in the Central African Republic in 1987, when our team member drowned, had taught me that it was always useful to have a safety net when travelling through new countries.

As it happened, I had heard of Alistair Bryant, the British defence attaché in Morocco, even though we hadn't met. He was several years younger, but fortunately also knew of me and suggested we meet up if I passed through Rabat. This was really convenient as I had a few days spare before meeting Tania and Millie and hoped Alistair would provide me with a secure place to park the wagon while I did some exploring. My general rule of thumb when in a city was to catch taxis, reducing the chances of having an accident or incident with the campervan.

I arrived in the capital city, which is about a two-hour drive south of Larache, and was instantly impressed. It's modern, very French and very clean and well swept. Alistair had given me directions to his house, but I was struggling with the Waze mobile app doing its best to guide me through streets mainly signposted in Arabic. Then, with frustration setting in as I was getting low on dopamine, I noticed a white woman and two children feeding a stray dog that had a litter of puppies. She was wearing smart slacks, a short-sleeved cotton shirt, headscarf and sunglasses. I knew instantly she was an army officer's wife. I wound down the van's window, about to ask if she was Emma Bryant, when she smiled and said, 'You must be Guy Deacon.'

No doubt the large Cure Parkinson's logo was a giveaway. And, just as I had met Mohammed's uncle completely by fluke a few days ago, fortune had smiled once again and I had found the Bryants. She pointed down the road. 'We live a couple of blocks away. I'll see you there in a moment.'

They had a magnificent house with a beautiful garden and two swimming pools. It was a reminder that defence attachés have a vital diplomatic role and need to look grand, as high-profile visitors always pass critical judgment on the lifestyles of different nations.

The Bryants treated me as a long-lost friend rather than an itinerant sponger and introduced me to their network of fellow defence attachés, including one from America who provided me with a month's worth of MRE (Meal Ready to Eat) military rations. It was a welcome break, and I felt thoroughly refreshed as I drove inland to meet my wife and daughter in Marrakesh.

Tania and Millie would be with me for two weeks. We headed for Imlil, a small village which felt like a quirky ski resort below Jebel Toubkal, the highest peak in northern Africa. There we stayed in a fine old castle that had been converted into a hotel, which would be our base for a week of trekking in the Atlas Mountains. Millie and Tania are extremely energetic and a hike with them on the slopes is certainly no walk in the park.

Although my Parkinson's was debilitating, by 2019 it had not yet reached stage three and I could still walk distances. I'm not an expert on gait, but it seems to me that we humans walk as if we are about to fall over. We lean forward and as the next move would be to land flat on our faces, we put a foot out to prevent that, and so on. As a Parkinson's sufferer, I take that to the extreme – I really am about to fall flat on my face and have to move my feet quickly, as though every step might be my last. This also means stopping is not straightforward and my momentum often results in bumping into walls, doors or people.

Despite that, I covered some fair distances that week and on most days trekked for close on ten miles. The way I walk meant going uphill was easier and on some downhill stretches our thoughtful guide would take me by the arm to stop me gaining speed and losing control.

Leaving the mountains, we drove west to Essaouira, a popular resort on Morocco's Atlantic coast where trade winds, known as *alizé*, are a magnet for surfers – whether board, wind or kite. Tania was already a top-class windsurfer and, although the waves weren't big, both she and Millie also learnt to surf with a board and rode horses along the sandy beaches in the warm winter sun. It was the perfect ending for a superb holiday and after celebrating new year, they flew home from Marrakesh.

However, if I'm completely honest, I prefer empty deserts to crowded beaches, and that would be exactly where I was heading next. For this I had the ideal partner, my old university friend David Attenburrow, who had been a fellow member of the Grand Erg Occidental expedition twenty-five years earlier. When I asked if he wanted to do another desert trip, this time in Morocco, he simply said, 'Yes please.'

I picked him up at Marrakesh airport and we headed south to the Erg Chebbi ('Sea of Dunes'), a thirty-one-mile stretch of sand dunes along the Algerian border that tower up to 1,200 feet and are among the tallest in the Sahara. We both wanted to relive past glories and we had no specific route, so we just undertook a general meander towards Western Sahara. We would travel when and where we pleased.

David is not only great fun, but as a bonus he's also technically skilled. He understands how things *really* work, knowing what a vehicle can do in extremely testing conditions and what might go wrong. Consequently, he is ready to give anything a go, but takes calculated risks.

We left Marrakesh at about 4 p.m., which meant crossing the Atlas Mountains at night – something not recommended in mid-winter with snowdrifts, high winds, icy roads and hairpin bends. But David's an extremely accomplished driver and we took it slowly, picking our way through some pretty hairy gorges with just headlights illuminating the way ahead. Eventually we descended onto a sandy plain as dawn was breaking, the rising sun shimmering on the vast desert in front and snow-capped peaks behind. It had been tricky at times, but intensely exhilarating.

The road was now as straight as an arrow, a welcome respite from snaking mountain passes and the van performed brilliantly as we headed for Erg Chebbi's largest dunes. The most critical thing to get right when driving in the desert is tyre pressure. Tyres require constant adjustment. Higher pressure is for gravel, lower pressure for sand, but surprisingly, dunes often rise out of gravel plains and consequently have hard ground surrounding them. As a result, you can be driving on soft sand one moment and compact gravel the next.

We were experimenting to see how far we could get on various pressures and had our tyres on 30 p.s.i. (pounds per square inch) when we came to the top of a shallow sandy ridge. Increasingly steep dunes stretched to the horizon and it looked as if the sand would be too soft to cross.

'I don't like it,' I said.

David nodded. 'No point in getting stuck for no reason.'

So we decided to act our age – wise, almost-60-year-olds rather than gung-ho youngsters – and were about to turn back to find another route when two Moroccans in a Land Cruiser drove up.

'Are you people all right?' the driver asked.

'We're absolutely fine,' I said. Then, pointing to the dunes ahead, I added, 'It's too difficult for this van. We're turning back.'

'No, you'll be OK,' the driver said. 'Just follow us.'

David and I looked at each other. Then shrugged – as I said, he's always willing to take a chance if the risks are acceptable. In this case, we were following locals with desert knowledge and if we did get stuck, the Toyota could hopefully pull us out.

'OK,' I said. 'We'll be right behind you.'

They introduced themselves as Omar and Hamid, then took off at a fair lick. We managed to keep up, but not for long. A few moments later, just as we started climbing the first proper dune, the van shuddered to a halt. We were stuck, and every spin of the wheels resulted in digging in deeper. Alarmingly, the van also started to tilt as the soft sand was on a slope. If we had continued there was a real risk of the wagon toppling onto its side and our only hope was that Omar and Hamid would be able to pull us out.

The Moroccans came back, got out of their truck, had a quick look at our predicament, then burst out laughing. 'Your tyres are too hard,' said one.

Indeed, in all the excitement of meeting our new friends, we had forgotten to deflate the tyres. They still were pumped to 30 p.s.i., way too high for sand and it was surprising that we'd got as far as we had. We quickly deflated them to 15 p.s.i., dug away as much sand as we could and reversed gingerly down the dune.

With the correct pressure, tyres float on the surface of the sand rather than dig in and soon we were on our way, with the van gliding over the desert with ease. The wagon far exceeded my expectations – it was not specifically designed for sand travel and we were loaded to the gunnels with tools, provisions and other kit. Yet it kept up with an unloaded Toyota that had been fitted with special dune tyres. From that moment on, I had total confidence that we could get through anything.

We followed Omar and Hamid to their desert workshop on the other side of the dunes for lunch. It turned out they were tour guides, providing visitors with a genuine desert experience in the Erg Chebbi and that evening they took us to one of their luxury desert campsites. Being mid-winter, there were no tourists, so we sat around a blazing wood fire while they played hand drums and smoked a bit of weed. Thinking I had overdone it with my giant spliff in Andorra and still eager to see if it helped my Parkinson's, I decided to give cannabis one more try. However, even a tiny amount prompted the same disastrous nausea and a complete inability to move, proving once and for all that marijuana doesn't work for me.

Next morning, we said goodbye to Omar and Hamid, who had gone out of their way for us – a hallmark of Morocco – and drove along the southern edge through stunning and challenging country towards Western Sahara. For the next week we lived like nomads, totally self-reliant and travelling where the whim took us. We slept under megawatt stars, wrapped warmly to ward off temperatures plummeting to well below zero, while meals were scooped out of cans and washed down with local beer. Even though we had GPS and a map, at times our exact position was an estimation. Other than stopping to eat, sleep, decant diesel from the jerry cans or take yet more photographs, we headed west seeing hardly anyone. It was exactly what I wanted – a slice of heaven.

Although we rarely mentioned Parkinson's, David sensed my deep frustration that I was no longer as strong as I used to be, often barely able to lift things and I had lost much of my dexterity. It was impossible not to notice how much slower I was, even with simple chores, and how much I now couldn't do. As a result, without speaking about it, he did a lot of the driving, set up rudimentary campsites at our overnight stops and prepared most of the meals.

But despite that, never once did his confidence in me waver. Never once did he mention that perhaps this trip – my odyssey – might be too much. His trust and confidence were vital, and the time we spent together in the desert will always be cherished.

After five days of travelling parallel to Algeria, we reached the main road which led to the Western Sahara border.

Except there wasn't one. We weren't aware that, as Morocco effectively controlled the disputed territory, there was, for all intents and purposes, no border. Originally known as Spanish Sahara, Spain handed over the country in 1975 to Morocco and Mauritania, who made joint claims. A war almost immediately broke out with the Polisario Front, a nationalist movement of the indigenous Sahrawi people, so Mauritania withdrew its claims. This left Morocco in control of 80 per cent of the territory, including all major cities and most of the natural resources. Today, two-thirds of the population is Moroccan and Morocco refers to Western Sahara as its southern provinces.

The largest city is Laayoune and sadly that was where David would leave me, flying back to England. It had been an extraordinary trip, a fascinating mix of sand dunes, rocks, Ergs and unmarked tracks in wild countryside that defies description.

Next stop would be Mauritania.

18

Mauritania

My amazing two weeks with David, travelling in some of the harshest country I had so far encountered, took more out of me than I realised.

Luckily for me, as David flew out of Laayoune, I bumped into Jon Felton, an ex-British Army corporal who was part of the UN Mission for the Referendum in Western Sahara (MINURSO). The UN has a small presence in the Western Sahara to keep a watchful eye on developments and ensure that the Sahrawi people are not discriminated against and Jon was chief logistics officer. I first met him ten years ago when I was with the UN's peacekeeping mission in the DRC and he had been based in Uganda. However, he says we go back even further, as he was with the Royal Corps of Transport in Germany during the 1980s and his unit had been responsible for moving our armoured vehicles around. At that time, I was leading the QDG's B Squadron in Sennelager but can't claim to remember him from those days. However, he was a typical British Army corporal: tough, reliable and so confident that he thinks he can do almost anything – which invariably means he can. He's just the guy you want on your side in an emergency.

I was not in an emergency situation, but he saw I was exhausted and immediately gave me the master room at his Laayoune flat to recover. He didn't know much about Parkinson's, but instinctively sensed what needed to be done: cooking easy to eat food, unobtrusively helping me when necessary and just being charming and very easy company.

Thanks to Jon, I soon was strong enough to travel again, and set off for Mauritania, which is pretty much down a dead-straight road along the Atlantic coast. There was not much to see, except for a beach resort called Dakhla, the southernmost point of Western Sahara. It's basically a windswept lagoon where a spit of sand separates shallow water from the ocean and is a mecca for mainly European wind and kitesurfers. There were lots of motorhomes and campervans and a clubhouse where the hordes of surfers congregated. Far too many, for my liking, and it reminded me of a beach near Chtouka in Morocco where I arrived thinking I was on my own only to discover an entire flotilla of French and German campervans had beaten me to it.

I spent a night before heading south, listening to music and knocking off the miles at my own pace without troubling anyone else. As mentioned, I'm not a fan of conventional campsites and finding somewhere solitary was my main goal when the sun set. I did this by simply turning off the road and driving at a right angle for about three miles, which I figured would be far enough away from other people. I would then wait for a while to see if I would be disturbed and if not, make something to eat. If anyone did appear, I moved off.

I never cooked as it was too fiddly to light a stove, prepare food, wash up and put utensils away. Instead, meals were always something simple – usually sardines on crackers or bread rolls washed down with a local beer. The fridge's sole purpose was to keep beers cold – something always important, but even more so in the desert.

I would then upload the best photos I had taken that day to Polarsteps. As the main aim of the journey was to raise awareness of Parkinson's, I had brought along two quality cameras to record the journey and illustrate regular progress reports. But what I hadn't bargained for was camera shake – thanks to my disease – not to mention the hassle of setting the cameras up, making sure batteries were charged, fannying about pressing buttons, trying to read settings in the failing light and cleaning out sand. Those chores take a few seconds for most people, but not if you have Parkinson's. Consequently, I soon found it far easier and just as effective to take pictures with my mobile phone using a selfie stick!

It was also difficult to upload posts to Polarsteps as, by the time I had set up camp, it was dark and my eyes were not what they used to be. Not having the motor skills to type accurately, I preferred to dictate posts which – with even a mild Parkinson's stammer – resulted in some extraordinary errors.

After sorting out the website, I would do rudimentary vehicle checks: tightening nuts and bolts and checking various bits of wire and anything else I needed to keep an eye on. My tools were perfectly organised in a stacking system that I designed myself. The bottom box stored heavy stuff like wooden blocks and bottle jacks, the next was packed with lighter tools, such as hammers and spanners, as well as oil and other lubricants and above that was the electrical kit, including loads of cable ties, string and tape. Good organisation was essential, as with Parkinson's even minor chores take twice as long to complete. For example, just getting a spanner to fit onto a bolt was an achievement. All of this was extremely time-consuming and I seldom got to bed before 11 p.m., or was ready to move the next morning by 10 a.m.

But the main benefit of travelling alone was that I could move at my own pace, trundling along merrily in my own little world. I didn't even have to clean my teeth if I didn't feel up to it and supper was often peanut butter spooned out of a jar.

The Mauritanian border post was in the middle of nowhere, a nondescript building with a car park in some sand dunes. One would have thought that a car park was superfluous in the world's third-largest desert, but not only was it compulsory to park there, you had to pay for the privilege of doing so. There were also fixers to help you get through, if you needed them. That was the theory, but in reality I didn't have a choice as the moment I stepped out of my vehicle a fixer snatched my passport and said, 'Follow me.' To compound the issue, border officials would only speak to the fixers, so DIY travellers stand no chance. But to give my fixer his due, he did make my life far easier by knowing which window to go to and which person to talk to.

However, I hadn't banked on using a fixer as I had checked on iOverlander, a useful free travel website, I had all the correct documentation and I was confident on getting through on my own. By the time I discovered that was almost impossible, it was too late. So when the fixer wanted payment for his services, I didn't have cash on me.

'No problem,' he said. 'I take you to cashpoint in Nouadhibou.'

I needed to do that anyway, as whenever I crossed a border my first priority was to get cash and a sim card for my phone. Both were vital: one to pay people like the fixer, the other to use for Waze and Google Maps navigation.

Nouadhibou, a fishing port and major railway siding for the country's iron ore exports, was several miles away. But to get there we had to cross what appeared to be a vision from a B-grade science fiction movie – a three-hundred-yard stretch of road strewn with thousands upon thousands of empty water bottles. As there were no rubbish bins, travellers simply tossed their junk out of the window. Driving over a thick carpet of crackling plastic gave added meaning to the word 'surreal'.

The fixer took me to three cashpoints in Nouadhibou. The first two didn't work, but fortunately the third – and final – one did. I got some cash but what I didn't know was that a few days beforehand Mauritania had devalued its currency – the ouguiya – by the simple expedient of knocking a zero off each denomination. If, like me, you didn't know what the exchange rate was with the euro, you were doubly confused. I had no idea of what I was paying the fixer and started haggling half-heartedly from a position of total weakness. Luckily – or so I thought at the time – another chap pitched up to help, and with a big smile introduced himself as Omaar. He spoke some English – in fact, he claimed he first approached me to practise his language skills – and said he would sort out the fixer.

That he did, then said I should stay with him and took me to his house, where I parked the wagon in a dirty street. He then hailed a taxi to take us around town to get various bits and pieces and have a meal and, although nothing seemed untoward, I was very aware that I was leaving the van unguarded in an area I knew nothing about. Fortunately, it was still there when we returned.

Omaar then invited me to come and meet a 'friend' and, before I knew it, a scantily clad woman looking remarkably like a sex worker climbed into the van. Not entirely surprising really, as that is what she turned out to be! I politely declined her offer whereas Omaar did not. That was fine with me (who was I to judge local practices?) although I was a little irked when Omaar asked me to pay her so she could go home. I had little option but to do as he requested or else risk a shouting match with an irate woman in the middle of the street. I knew he was ripping me off, which was fine to some extent, but this was going too far.

The next day Omaar asked if I wanted to see some shipwrecks. I thought he would take me to see some old Arab dhows, so reluctantly agreed and ended up having to pay a beach guard wads of unknown cash to park the wagon and look at what turned out to be rusting relics of commercial vessels stranded inshore. This, I later learnt, was the 'famous' Nouadhibou ships' graveyard.

However, he had one more scam up his sleeve. As I was driving him home, he suddenly said, 'Stop, you've been caught speeding.' I saw some policemen in my rear view mirror, but wasn't sure if they had actually stopped me. It certainly didn't look like it. And I was pretty sure I was not speeding – certainly no more than other traffic around me.

'Give me money and I'll pay them off,' he said.

I handed over another wedge of ouguiya. I had no idea of how much but by now considered anything would be cheap to get rid of Omaar. As far as I could gather, he did pay the police something.

Omaar was the only person who had blatantly taken advantage of me, but to give him credit, he had been good company and was rather funny about it all. However, the 'speeding' incident was the final straw. I kicked him out of the car and continued heading south towards the capital city, Nouakchott. It was a long drive through rolling desert, although there were by now some signs of vegetation. The biggest change was that it was getting much hotter and very quickly.

Although Nouakchott is the nerve centre of the country, as far as I could make out the only remarkable feature was that virtually every second car was a Mercedes-Benz C-Class. No doubt these upmarket vehicles once belonged to wealthy Europeans, but either through legitimate imports or smuggling rings, had dodged first world scrapheaps and found their way to one of the globe's poorer countries for a new lease of life. It's rather ironic that in a country where 42 per cent of the population live in dire poverty, the most common car is a Mercedes.

However, I do have one good thing to say about Mauritania; their chocolate sandwiches are out of this world. This may sound incongruous – bread and chocolate – but the way the Mauritanians do it is absolutely delicious. A highlight of my day was stopping at a roadside *duka*, stall, and buying a hunk of freshly baked bread dripping with rich chocolate.

There were several crossings from Mauritania into Senegal and one I was warned to steer clear of was the Rosso border post, about which I'd heard numerous horror stories of chaos and corruption. The most common story is of travellers being stranded halfway across the bridge on the River Senegal, unable to go back to Mauritania and unable to proceed to Senegal unless they pay a bribe.

I decided to cross at the Diama border control, close to the Atlantic coast, which involved a drive through a remote nature reserve. The road was a rutted berm and I didn't see much wildlife; just some flamingos, a couple of warthogs and a solitary baboon. Most of the excitement involved swerving off the berm to avoid speeding lorries. I decided not to use a fixer at this border post, so it took longer but was still easy to buy a Senegalese visa.

As I crossed the river, I also crossed an ethnic divide. I was now in Black Africa.

19

Senegal

My first stop in Senegal was Saint-Louis, a town at the mouth of the Senegal River and a UNESCO World Heritage Site. It was once an important trading hub, but today is better known as a cultural tourist centre. Many of the historic French colonial buildings are now hotels.

And that's exactly where I was heading, the hotels, which is what I usually do when arriving in a new city, as that's where there's free parking. One of the first hotels I saw was the de La Poste, which was perfect as not only could I park the wagon, but I was allowed to use the hotel's swimming pool. This was always welcome, as for Parkinson's sufferers, a swimming pool is ideal for bathing, even though one can't use soap. With our impaired balance, it's very easy to slip and fall in a shower and extremely difficult to get up. Consequently, whenever I am able to jump into a swimming pool, I do so with delight.

Equally good was my first cold beer in an air-conditioned bar for almost a week – an excellent local brew called La Gazelle.

Knowing my van was secure, I went sightseeing in the historic city, which was once the capital of both Senegal and Mauritania in colonial days, before I turned in for the night. The strong French influence was a welcome change from the drabness of Nouakchott.

The next afternoon I set off for Dakar, almost two hundred miles south. One of the great pleasures of travelling in Africa is how dramatically everything around you changes, both culturally and ecologically, as if watching a movie. For example, the further south I travelled through Morocco, rolling sand dunes replaced snow-capped mountains for as far as the eye could see. Then in Mauritania, the vast dunes gradually evolved into shrubs and small bushes, usually thorny acacias. This was the Sahara transforming into the Sahel, the change from desert to savannah. The bushes got bigger as I approached Senegal, merging into wooded areas after crossing the border. Of course, once in the two Guineas, Sierra Leone, and Gabon, it was mainly tropical forests.

The people also visibly changed, with the Arabs and Berbers in the north gradually giving way to sub-Saharan Africans. This meant stunning cultural diversity, the most noticeable being food and music. I'm not a great foodie and don't eat out much – the highlight was Mauritanian chocolate sandwiches – but I always downloaded local music. It differs vastly, from the haunting *chaabi* street songs in the souks of North Africa to the *mbalax* of Senegal, a fusion of traditional and pop, and the Afrobeat of Nigeria, a combination of traditional West African folk, American funk and jazz.

I had already organised accommodation in Dakar as a good friend from my Durham University days, Hugh Davies, had put me in touch with Victor Ndiaye, who lived in the Senegalese capital. I had phoned Victor from the UK and when he heard that I knew Hugh, he invited me to stay. Unfortunately, due to bad timing, I arrived in this bustling city of more than a million people in late afternoon peak traffic. Also, in West Africa, most major cities are on the coast, which means the setting sun shines directly into your eyes, making navigation with a humble phone app even more of a nightmare than necessary.

Despite the manic traffic and being half-blinded, I managed to find Victor's house, in a gated community and, as his wife and kids were away, there was plenty of room. The only other person was Tattie, Victor's aunt from France, who spent most summers in Dakar. She was eighty but had the energy of someone half her age and was great company. My conversational French was improving dramatically, although Tattie's rapid-fire delivery was challenging at times. However, we got along famously and, as Victor was often away on business trips, she was my constant companion.

Victor was very well connected and generously offered to sort out my visas for my next two destinations, Guinea-Bissau and Guinea. That was quite a weight off my shoulders and I filled in a lot of forms, handed over my passport and the wait began. I expected to be staying with Victor for about a week until all my documentation was sorted out, blissfully unaware that Africa moves at its own pace.

Whenever Victor was away, he put his chauffer Fred at our disposal and I saw a lot of the city with Tattie and his Senegalese sister-in-law Miriam, who knew the city intimately. One of the highlights was visiting Ngor, a quaint, tiny island in the Bay of Dakar that's crammed with bijoux cafés and bars. It's about a ten-minute *pirogue* – a small boat – ride from the mainland and I had never heard of it before. But what made it special for me – and every Francophone – is that France Gall lived there until she died in 2018. Although barely known in the UK, she was a legendary *yé-yé* singer, a lively French style of pop music (based on the 'yeah-yeah' Beatles era), and a Eurovision contest winner. I loved her songs when I was based in Germany and jumped at the chance to visit her island home.

Noticing my interest in music, Tattie and Miriam also took me to a rock concert starring Senegalese superstar Wasis Diop. Although his sound is somewhat heavy and I won't be buying his albums, it was a magical evening made even more so by the eclectic mixture of people of all colours, classes and statuses having a great time dancing and singing. I found myself thinking that we British who believe East Africa is the continent's crown jewel might be wrong. Looking at West Africa, I know where I would rather spend time.

Another impressive spectacle is the African Renaissance Monument, a 171-foot bronze statue on top of one of the twin hills known as Collines des Mamelles in Dakar. Overlooking the Atlantic Ocean, it's the tallest statue in Africa and the second-largest sculpture in the world. Despite much negative comment and the controversial building costs of £16.6 million, it's a popular tourist attraction – although at the time I was the only person there – with a platform inside the statue's head providing panoramic views of the city. This was the first of my four bucket list African sites – the others being the Basilica at Yamoussoukro, the Matadi suspension bridge spanning the Congo River and the Rorke's Drift battlefield in South Africa, where eleven Victoria Crosses were awarded.

I also had lunch with my former DRC peacekeeping mission boss, now retired, General Babacar Gaye and his wife Mame Diara. He was most charming and appeared to have forgotten that I once used unilaterally 'mission command' to bypass political problems with the Indian and Pakistani peacekeeping forces. I had sent him an email before leaving the UK warning that I planned to drive down Africa through Senegal and he said I should look him up. Even so, I think he was surprised to see me, but it was a great reunion.

The kindness of strangers that I had encountered so often on this trip continued to astonish me. By now, after almost a hundred days on the road – or more accurately gravel and sand – the wagon needed servicing and I took it to a garage recommended by Victor. It was owned by Alain Monteiro, a mechanic who worked in Saly, a seaside resort south of Dakar. He and his team spent several hours checking and fixing various things, so when he handed me the bill I expected a fairly hefty hit on my wallet. Instead, I was shocked at how small it was – a fraction of what I was expecting.

When I questioned him, he asked almost apologetically, 'Is it too much?' He knew my trip was about Parkinson's and obviously wanted to help in the best way he could.

'Not too much,' I replied. 'It's far too little.' I insisted on paying more, but it still in no way reflected the amount of quality work he had done. The genuine goodness in so many people is extraordinary.

However, reality hit home soon afterwards when I was about to turn onto the road ten yards from Alain's garage and several gendarmes ran over, waving me down. They claimed I wasn't wearing a seatbelt, despite the fact that it was clearly obvious I was in the process of buckling up and wasn't even on the main road. This was purely a scam to fleece tourists.

I replied in English, shaking my head and saying I didn't understand what they were getting at. As they became increasingly hostile, I picked up my phone. General Gaye had told me over lunch to call him if I ran into any problems. So I thought, Right, you bastards. I'm going to ring your boss. General Gaye picked up almost immediately. 'General, I don't have a problem yet,' I said, 'but just thought I would touch base with you in case it does become a problem.'

When the gendarmes heard me speak French, they realised they had been beaten. They also knew I had stronger friends than they had and quickly let me go.

However, another drama was looming on the horizon. I had now been in Senegal for almost four weeks and my visas for Guinea-Bissau and Guinea still had not come through. I was also becoming uncomfortable about overstaying my welcome with Victor, although I knew this was not a major problem for him as the house was largely empty. But I am always mindful of abusing people's hospitality.

However, there was not much I could do, as I couldn't go anywhere without a visa. That's the name of the game – and it was to some extent a game. Travelling overland down Africa is like playing snakes and ladders, except that there are three times as many snakes. Just when you think you're making progress climbing a ladder, everything goes wrong and you slide down a snake.

It is therefore really important to relax and accept that Africa often marches to a different drumbeat. Enjoy the game, no matter how long the snakes and how short the ladders, rather than fret about situations you cannot control. Otherwise, you will go mad.

But for me these delays had an added consequence. My Parkinson's medication was in danger of running out.

The thought filled me with dread.

20

The Gambia

Let's face it: without treatment I would not have been able to attempt this odyssey. I simply couldn't undertake the physical task without medication to assist muscle control and combat depression, fatigue and anxiety. That's the reality of Parkinson's.

In a nutshell, the disease is caused by low levels of a chemical in the brain called dopamine, which causes tremors, spasms and poor motor skills. That's the medical description, but it nowhere near describes how much the disease hampers one's mobility. Simply leaning on the side of a vehicle can sometimes be a tricky balancing act, while there are times you just lie on the floor without the will or the energy to get up. On top of this, there are many occasions when you can't speak properly and stuttering sounds rather than words come out of your mouth. Consequently, I take one Pramipexole and six Sinemet tablets a day to boost dopamine levels and help make life bearable for as long as possible.

To cross Africa overland is an extreme adventure for even the fit and healthy, let alone someone with a debilitating sickness and now my supply of tablets was running low. I would pick up another month's supply that had been posted to me from the UK when I reached Sierra Leone, but it did mean I needed to speed up my journey.

However, that was the last thing I wanted to do, as I had no intention of having my African odyssey defined by the number of pills I needed. That was the antithesis of my goal – so much so that I was now seriously considering extending the journey all the way to the southernmost tip of the continent. One reason for this was that I had raised a bit of money for Cure Parkinson's through a JustGiving page, and my Polarsteps blog already 'boasted' seventy-six followers. That's obviously nowhere near celebrity status, but it indicated genuine interest in what I was doing. I reckoned that if I could get more than a hundred followers, that would be enough to justify adjusting my travel plans and carry on going south.

To be on the safe side, I started cutting down on my meds, which meant I had longer periods of being slower both physically and mentally. I also started looking around to see if I could buy pills in Senegal. I first had to find a doctor who would give me a prescription, then a pharmacy able to deliver. It wasn't cut and dried by any means. In fact, it took me three or four days just to find a source. The medication was also exorbitant and that more than anything else hammered home how difficult life was for Parkinson's sufferers in Africa. If I struggled to find prescription pills in a modern Francophone city with shopping malls, gated communities, boutique hotels and restaurants, imagine how hard it would be for people in the back of beyond.

Part of my ambassadorial responsibilities for Cure Parkinson's was to do rudimentary research into neurological care in Africa while passing through various countries. I decided now to also focus on the availability of Parkinson's medication – or, as I was fast finding out, the lack thereof.

Eventually my visas came through and I set off for Guinea-Bissau, but first had to pass through The Gambia, the only country in the world with a capital 'The' in its name. It was sad to say goodbye to Victor, Tattie and Miriam, whose hospitality and generosity had been immense and I sincerely hoped I hadn't overstayed my welcome.

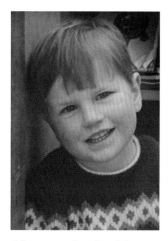

Me, aged four, in 1965, when life was simple.

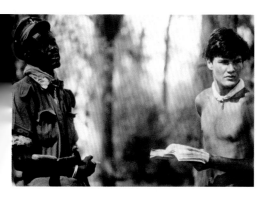

On my first expedition to northern Kenya in 1982. Here a local militia man is seeking payment having deterred an attack by cattle raiders from the Ethiopian border.

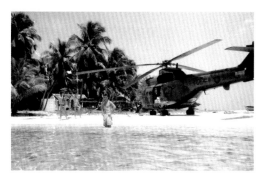

A tough life: visiting a remote observation post, where British soldiers were monitoring Guatemalan vessels from the southernmost caye of Belize, in 1989.

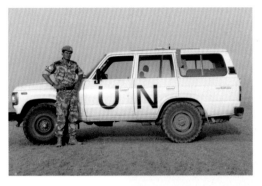

In Iraq and Kuwait in 1991, after the First Gulf War, free to roam the desert before the UN wrote the rule book.

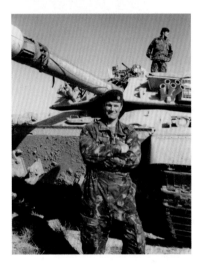

In Canada with my tank in 1999, while commanding B Squadron.

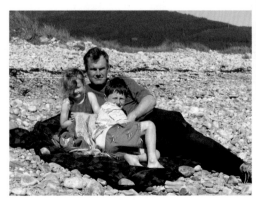

Another holiday in Scotland with Millie and Wilfred, near Brora in Sutherland, 2002.

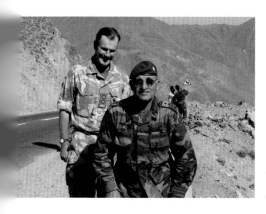

With General Karimi in
Afghanistan, in 2005.

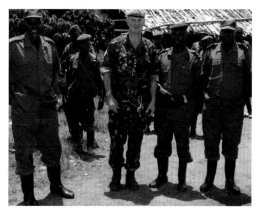

Visiting outposts with the leaders of the FARDC, the Armed Forces of the
Democratic Republic of the Congo, in the DRC in 2010.

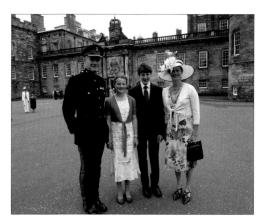

About to receive my OBE,
in 2011, on my return from
the DRC, at Holyrood
Palace, Edinburgh, with
Millie, Wilfred and Tania.

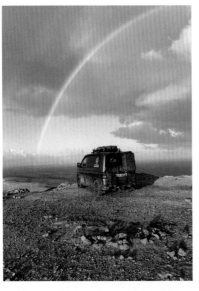

Following the coast through Morocco.

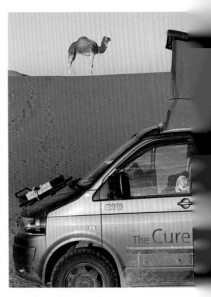

A morning visitor in the Sahara.

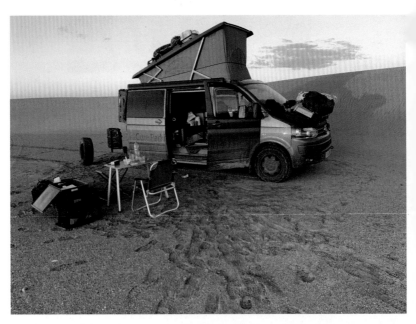

A typical campsite, tucked behind a dune, in Morocco.

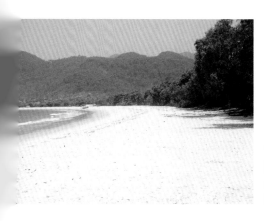

Tokeh Beach, south of Freetown, in Sierra Leone, reputedly one of the most beautiful in the world.

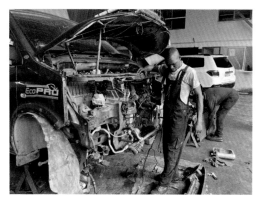

The shocking sight of the wagon in Abidjan, Côte d'Ivoire, waiting for the new clutch to arrive.

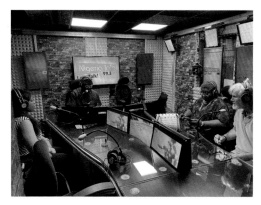

One of the many radio interviews I did, this time with Omotola Thomas and Morin Desalu in Lagos, Nigeria.

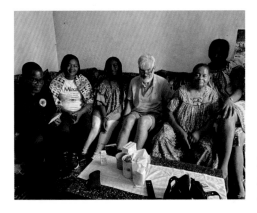

Meeting people with Parkinson in Yaoundé, Cameroon, with Hilaire Roger (far left).

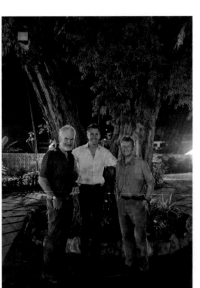

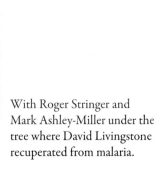

In Lagos, Nigeria, with Tim Hepburn and Omotola Thomas.

With Roger Stringer and Mark Ashley-Miller under the tree where David Livingstone recuperated from malaria.

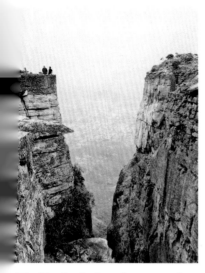

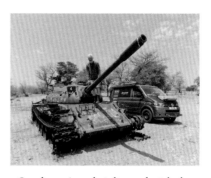

Southern Angola is littered with the debris of war. Here a Russian T62 tank reminds us of this country's turbulent past.

The Tundavala Gap, about ten miles north-west of Lubango, in Angola, where both UNITA and the MPLA used to throw prisoners to their deaths.

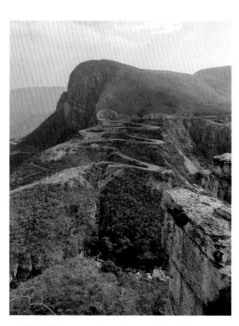

The wonderful 'Precipice' road towards Lubango, in Angola.

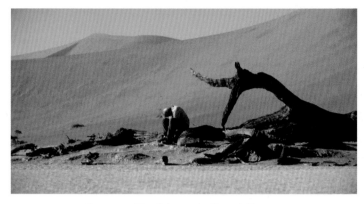

Resting at Deadvlei in the Namib Desert.

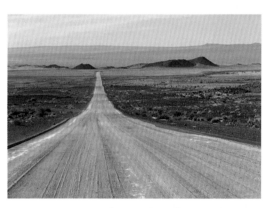

Vast and empty Namibia.

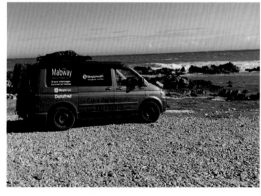

Finally at Cape Agulhas, Africa's southernmost point.

However, potential disaster struck a couple of hours later when I glanced in my rear view mirror to see clouds of smoke billowing from the back of the wagon. None of my dashboard warning lights were flashing but, even so, I pulled over into a layby to check it out. I couldn't see anything wrong, so the only way to determine if I had a serious problem was to get the bash plate off for a closer look. I jacked up the vehicle and with much difficulty wrangled the hefty slab of metal off the vehicle's underbelly.

Wriggling my hand inside, I instantly felt something wet. Surprisingly, it was water. I was expecting leaking oil or something equally ominous after what had happened to the diff in Andorra. Then it dawned. The smoke was steam caused by condensation from the vehicle's air conditioners dripping onto the hot exhaust system. I had gone through all that grimy hassle for no reason at all.

Even worse, I now had to put it all back together. It was dark, which may be my favourite time to travel, but not for carrying out mechanical repairs. By reverse engineering with jacks, blocks and military-grade cursing, I managed to fit the bash-plate bolts onto the chassis. Next job was to tighten the nuts, somewhat difficult with my poor motor skills, as just aligning the spanner is a formidable task – particularly with only a torch beam to guide me.

I would like to say I completed the job myself, but after I had been under the wagon for about four hours, a roadside recovery man arrived and asked if he could help.

'No thanks,' I said. 'I'm managing.' I was determined not to give up.

He crouched down, looked at what I was doing, and smiled. 'I think you do need my help.'

I sighed. Sweat was dripping off me like a hot shower. He was right. I handed him the spanner and it took him a few minutes to tighten the bolts and I was ready to go.

The Gambia is completely surrounded by Senegal except for a fifty-mile stretch of Atlantic coastline on its western extremity.

The country is the smallest on the African mainland – slightly less than the total area of Jamaica – and juts inland like a rudely extended finger for 295 miles on either side of the Gambia River. Its widest inland point is only thirty miles.

I was advised by the iOverlander app to cross the river, turn right and head west for the capital Banjul once I crossed the border. That's what I did and was driving along happily when a policeman stopped me. 'Where are you going?' he asked.

'Banjul.'

'Why are you on this road?'

'Isn't it the right road?'

He shook his head. 'The other road on the north bank is much better and faster.'

He then advised me to turn back north over the river and head for a village called Barra, where I would again cross the river and the capital was on the southern bank. I believed him and it seemed he had given me good advice. The road was excellent and with hardly any traffic, I rapidly approached Barra.

The only problem, I noticed as I arrived, was that there was no bridge across the river to Banjul. In fact, the only way to the capital city was to catch a ferry, with a timetable that seemed haphazard at best. I was told the boat would leave in about two hours – maybe – so there was nothing to do but wait. I was the only car there, but a lot of pedestrians were starting to queue up.

Then, just as the ferry was about to depart, cars started arriving from every direction. Scores of them – so many that we were ushered on board with barely inches separating each vehicle. I had to fold my wing mirrors to prevent them from being crushed. More alarmingly, all drivers had to remain in their cars as there was not enough space to open a door. If the ferry sank, it wouldn't be the captain going down with his ship – it would be us in our vehicles. Just as I had imagined tabloid newspaper stories recording my demise after smoking a spliff in Andorra, I envisioned a headline: 'Hundreds drowned and former English colonel missing in African tragedy.'

Fortunately, that didn't happen, although, as with most Parkinson's sufferers, death holds no real fear for me. We might have been packed like sardines and the ferry old and decrepit, but like much else in Africa, it still worked. Half an hour later I was in Banjul.

My hosts in the capital were Kamal and Mandi, who are among the most wonderful people I've met on my travels. They did not know me from a bar of soap – which I clearly needed when I arrived – but invited me to come and stay with them on the strength of an off-the-cuff request from a friend of a friend. I just wanted a place to park my van where I could sleep and asked if I could do so outside a restaurant they owned. But Kamal said it was also a discotheque that got a bit noisy at night, so I should rather park at their house.

Although ethnically Lebanese, Kamal is effectively Gambian while Mandi's family come from Sierra Leone. There are an estimated 300,000 Lebanese in West Africa, and most have been there for multiple generations. The first immigrants arrived in the early nineteenth century, fleeing oppression and an economic crisis in the Ottoman Empire and initially set up market stalls as small traders. Most settled in the Ivory Coast, the Côte d'Ivoire, where they make up ten per cent of the population in the city of Abidjan. But all West African countries have significant Lebanese diasporas and there is little doubt that their contribution to their adopted countries is immense.

I spent four days with Kamal and Mandi and they treated me like family, going for walks on beautiful beaches and feasting at their excellent restaurant, Kaya, which reminded me of a Bob Marley song and album by the same name. Compared to Senegal, The Gambia is very British, with English the official language and I found it a delightful country, not just because I'm a Brit.

Whenever I travel to anywhere new, I like to visit Commonwealth war grave cemeteries and pay my respects as an ex-soldier to those who have fallen for their country (or in some cases for somebody else's country). During the Second World War, Banjul – then called Bathurst – was an important British naval base and a vital stopover for convoys bound for the Middle East, India, South Africa and South America. The Commonwealth War Graves Commission site there is known as the Fajara War Cemetery and has 203 graves, of which four are still unidentified. I always find the tombstones mask some very moving stories and one in Fajara that particularly struck me was the final resting place of Tom R. Lewis, a cadet in the Merchant Navy on the ship MV *Deido*. He lies alongside a small number of other Brits and Canadians, but mainly soldiers serving with a Gambian regiment that was part of the West African Frontier Force.

The information chiselled onto the gravestone merely states that Tom Lewis died on 17 August 1945 – three months after the Germans surrendered – and that he came from Barry in Glamorgan, South Wales, not far from where I grew up as an army brat.

He was just seventeen.

It was time to move on. Heading south, I crossed back from The Gambia into Senegal for the 113-mile stretch to the Guinea-Bissau border.

21

Driving on the Wrong Side

I didn't need to go to Guinea-Bissau, a former Portuguese colony with a history of political instability and one of the lowest GDPs in the world. I could easily have turned inland and entered its far larger neighbour, the former French colony of Guinea. To distinguish between the two countries that both have the same name, Bissau, the capital, is suffixed.

However, hugging the Atlantic coast added to the integrity of my journey and, besides, I had never been there and thought it would be interesting. It's also famed for beautiful beaches. I had a more mundane reason as I was running low on cash and needed to get to an ATM rather urgently.

Once I had crossed the border, I turned off the main road and headed west for a coastal village called Varela. The main road was little more than a potholed track with a thin tarmac veneer and the route to the coast even worse. To head west you either needed to be a good dirt road driver or have a four-wheel drive. It's a four-hour trip with lots of red dust but worth every minute as, just past the village, lurks an idyllic deserted beach with a gently lapping warm sea and palm trees growing up to the dunes. A spit of fine white sand separates a lagoon where pelicans float next to waterlilies and dozens of songbirds break the otherwise golden silence.

I was the only person there and, after a refreshing dip in the ocean, made myself comfortable for the night. It was paradise and, unusually, I slept solidly for six hours.

But the next morning reality hit hard. For the first time on this trip, I felt utterly crippled by Parkinson's. I managed to have a lethargic swim and some breakfast – Mandi had made sure I had plenty of food before leaving Banjul – but despite my best efforts I was moving slower than a tortoise. Just getting dressed was a series of stilted lurches. I hoped it was simply a one-off bad day, a result of being frugal with meds to make sure I didn't run out before my resupply in Sierra Leone, but something told me it was more serious than that.

I managed to get going again and headed towards Bissau but to add to my debilitation, the wagon started making an ominous clunking sound. Again, there were no warning lights flashing, but I suspected it might be the long-suffering suspension starting to remind me that I was driving through some pretty wild country. It didn't affect the handling of the vehicle, but I had to be extra cautious going over potholes and bumps, which were the norm rather than exception on these roads. This meant going slower with more gear changes and even greater concentration, placing increasing demands on the dopamine sloshing around inside me.

I had no plans to explore Bissau; my sole purpose of stopping was to draw cash. It was dusk when I arrived, so I decided to camp outside the city and go in early next morning. At about 1 a.m. I woke and drove into Bissau's central business district, which was surreal beyond belief. There was not a single light shining in the entire city – no street lamps, neon advertising or even a traffic light. The only illumination was the odd torch flash from a security guard. I could almost hear Michael Jackson singing 'Thriller' in the background. With the help of my trusty iOverlander app, I found a cashpoint in a bank foyer where the security guard let me in. I keyed in my card details, grabbed the cash and left as hurriedly as I could.

The next day was plain sailing on good murram roads through what had clearly once been beautiful country, but now very much deforested with more dead tree stumps than canopy. Just before the Guinea border I had a flat tyre and it couldn't have happened at a worse time – my dopamine levels were falling and exhaustion was setting in. It was not an actual puncture – instead, the rim had been bent out of shape on another unavoidable pothole, quickly deflating the tyre. Each wheel weighed 88 pounds and the spare was mounted at chest height on the back door of the van, so it was not easy to lift on and off.

While psyching myself up to change the wheel, a small crowd of folk, either after a reward or genuinely trying to help, gathered around. Being positively minded, I assumed the latter and I was right. For them, this was the big event of the day in their village and in no time helpers were delving into the wagon to get out a jack and wheel spanners. It was all I could do to keep an eye on the van with prying fingers everywhere while trying to supervise the actual wheel change. I also had to hammer the bent steel wheel back into shape.

That night I camped at a petrol station and was minding my own business when several men in untidy uniforms approached, asking what I was doing. Thinking they were going to tell me to move on, I resignedly stopped assembling my bed and stepped out of the van. I asked, 'Are you police or army?'

The leader pointed to his uniform. 'Army.'

I smiled. 'I was a soldier once.'

Their whole demeanour changed. I was one of them, not just a traveller. I showed them a photo in uniform to prove that the old git in a scruffy T-shirt was a former military man. There were smiles all round. 'You can stay here and we will protect you,' the leader said.

I had deliberately brought several uniformed photos, looking the part in my former glory, so to speak, and they were invaluable. The respect that engendered was instant, showing that soldiers have a tight universal bond no matter where they come from.

The border crossing into Guinea was routine. It must have been, as I have absolutely no recollection of it.

But what I do remember is the clunking noise in the wagon getting significantly worse. The vehicle was still handling well, but whenever I asked anyone if there was a garage nearby, the answer was, 'No.' I had looked underneath for any loose items or obvious problems but to no avail. There was little I could do, except continue carefully.

Once in Guinea, I decided to head straight for the Sierra Leone border as I had no desire to drive into the capital Conakry. I'd heard the traffic was terrible and cities seething with humanity don't interest me much in any event. The route itself was straightforward – almost a direct line down the country – but the driving certainly wasn't. The clunking noise got worse and every third vehicle hogging the road was a massive logging truck loaded to the brim with giant tree trunks. Just as bad was dodging the plethora of Peugeot 504 taxis crammed with passengers and at least four feet of stuff strapped onto roof racks, and all seemingly driven by lunatics. This was exacerbated in the villages where scores of pedestrians also thronged haphazardly on the roads.

In one village a policeman stopped me and asked for a lift. It's always advisable to say, 'Yes,' in such instances, not least as you know you will get through the next roadblock without hassles. In this case he was doubly useful as I needed to get some dollars to buy a visa for Sierra Leone, saving weeks of waiting at an embassy. It had to be dollars as the customs control wouldn't accept any other currency. My new best friend, the policeman, guided me to a market and introduced me to a trader who would exchange West African CFA francs for dollars.

Arriving at the Pamelap border crossing into Sierra Leone I was initially impressed. It looked fairly well organised. All was going well as I checked out of Guinea and I was just finishing the process of getting into Sierra Leone when an official looked at the wagon and suddenly said, 'You can't go in.'

I stared back at her, confused. 'Why not?'

'Your car. It's a right-hand drive.'

Nowhere had I heard that you could not drive a right-hand vehicle in Sierra Leone. On the contrary, I thought it would be the opposite as the country was a former British colony, unlike most of West Africa which is francophone. But the woman was adamant; I could go no further.

'OK,' I said, not sure what to do next. 'How am I going to solve this problem?'

'I don't know. But you have to have permission from the minister of transport.'

When Sierra Leone decided to change to driving on the right, in accordance with the rest of West Africa, they had banned ownership of all right-hand drive vehicles. Being a former British colony, there were a lot of them, so the confusion that caused must have been immense. But only months before my arrival, they had taken it a step further, banning any right-hand drive vehicle unless specifically permitted by the Department of Transport.

As an army man, I plan for most eventualities, particularly unexpected ones. But this was a total sucker punch. I had absolutely no idea what to do next. I was unable to go back to Guinea as I had checked out and unable to go forward. I was well and truly stuck in no man's land.

Fortunately, the head of immigration at the border post, who introduced herself as Juliet, was as helpful as anyone could be under the circumstances and assigned a policeman called Sadi to assist me. Sadi drove me on the back of his motorbike to the licensing office in the next village, where they merely confirmed what Juliet had said. I then got hold of the British high commission in Freetown who also basically said I was stuck. No permit, no entry.

I decided to appeal for the sympathy vote. Turning to Juliet, I said, 'Look, I'm an old man and I'm a bit sick. I'm writing a daily blog on my travels and it will be sad if I said that despite coming all this way to a former British colony, I wasn't allowed in. And to have a poor, sick man having to spend his time stuck in no man's land – maybe that's not a good idea?' I had said it semi-tongue in cheek, trying to make the point that the border staff perhaps should try a little harder on my behalf.

It had the exact opposite effect. In spades. As soon as I mentioned the word 'sick', the border post staff sprang into action. They instantly ordered me to sit in a corner of the room and evacuated the building as if there were a bomb scare.

'What's going on?' I asked, stunned.

'You're contagious. We have to keep everyone away.'

Then it dawned. I knew that Covid-19 was spreading through Europe, but having been out of touch for so long was unaware that Africa was now also on high alert. Consequently, when I said I was sick, they immediately thought I was referring to the pandemic. 'No, no!' I said. 'Not Covid at all. I have Parkinson's.' I pointed to my van outside with the Cure Parkinson's logo. 'I'm doing this trip to raise awareness of Parkinson's disease, which I have. Not Covid.'

They were still really twitchy, but at least they were listening to me. 'You don't have Covid?' asked Juliet.

'No,' I repeated. 'Parkinson's. Nothing to do with Covid. In fact, for the last few weeks I've been on my own in my vehicle. I've been self-isolating.'

Luckily, Juliet had heard of Parkinson's, which is not always a given in Africa. I explained the symptoms to her, and the entire border control staff relaxed visibly.

'OK, you can stay here for the night in the car park,' she said. 'We'll see what we can do tomorrow.'

I returned to the wagon, roasting under the equatorial sun and being eaten alive by a swarm of mosquitoes as well as worrying like hell what was going to happen next. I quickly took pills before the situation spun out of control.

The following day I spoke to John Harper, the assistant defence attaché at the British high commission (the equivalent of an embassy in Commonwealth countries), while Juliet and her people at the border post spoke to their bosses. The end result was an agreement to allow me to drive to the high commission offices in Freetown and leave the wagon there, but to go no further without written permission from the minister of transport. I would have to attempt to get the right paperwork for that as soon as possible.

So, after nearly forty-eight hours, I was in Sierra Leone. Juliet and Sadi were probably as relieved to see the back of me as I was to be on the road again. But not for long. Three miles later I was stopped at a police checkpoint and sent back to the border by an officious rozzer who knew the law but not my circumstances. Juliet got extremely irritated with him, and I was on my way again, mindful that other police roadblocks would also probably turn me back. I had no option but to risk it.

Luckily, I wasn't stopped and the excellent road to Freetown was largely devoid of traffic, until about forty-five minutes from the capital when I hit peak traffic. And at sunset. Once again I was entering a big city in rush hour, navigating on a tiny mobile with the sun in my eyes. Even worse, my phone was running out of power.

Thankfully, I found the embassy without too much difficulty, arriving at about 9 p.m., and was met by John Harper, who had been so helpful in getting the minister of transport to allow me to drive to the high commission.

I was feeling completely knackered. And, worryingly, I knew it was more than just exhaustion. The past few days taking reduced dosages of pramipexole and Sinemet, combined with stress, heat and mosquitoes, had taken their toll with a vengeance.

'John, has a parcel arrived for me from the UK?' I asked.

He looked at me askance. 'Parcel?'

'Some pills,' I replied. 'For Parkinson's.'

He shook his head. All the hassles about right-hand drive vehicles and travel permits faded. I now had a far bigger problem.

I really needed those pills.

22

Covid

As I was several thousand miles from home, getting Parkinson's medication authorised in the UK proved to be difficult. In this case I was to blame, as having just retired from the Army, I still hadn't got to grips with civilian life and had not yet registered at a local doctor's surgery. This meant I couldn't simply get a prescription over the phone.

Instead, I had to get my friend Chris Forrest – whose mother had unhesitatingly allowed me to stay in her house in Limoges – to fetch a prescription from my neurologist in Edinburgh. Chris did all the legwork and then posted a month's supply to me at the British high commission in Sierra Leone. I am always staggered at the lengths good people will go to help those in need.

But even so, in those deeply uncertain times with Covid-19 lockdowns, I was not sure when – or if – the pills would arrive. In the interim, I had to ration myself, which resulted in my bad balance and already slow movements becoming even more exaggerated.

I also needed to get local money, as I was fast running out of cash. The exchange rate at the time was something like 7,600 Leones to one American dollar, which meant that a bundle of notes would buy precious little. One of the more frustrating tasks for Parkinson's sufferers is trying to extract a bank note from a wallet. In Europe, and to a lesser extent Morocco, this was not an issue as I used contactless debit cards, but the further south one travelled, the more cash was king. The locals could count hundreds of Leones in a millisecond, whereas I laboriously had to thumb each note. It would be bad enough if I were familiar with the currency, but with Parkinson's it was an excruciatingly slow process and struggling with an open wallet stuffed with notes can put anyone in an extremely vulnerable position.

Now finally allowed in the country, I parked at the British high commission for a few days, but the embassy obviously didn't want me to squat on their premises indefinitely and moved me to the International Military Assistance and Training Team (IMATT) compound. This was where British soldiers training the Sierra Leonean army stayed and, to my surprise, it was located in an area known as Leicester Square. It looked nothing like London's famed entertainment hub, but I soon found that many Freetown streets and squares are named after English cities and abolitionists such as William Wilberforce and Thomas Clarkson. Although the transatlantic slave trade was one of the most wretched periods in human history, at least Britain led the way in abolishing it – something I found that more West Africans than Britons appeared to be aware of today.

Then I got a pleasant surprise. I had not known that Alex Wilkinson, son of my friends Caroline and Henry, was in Freetown. His grandmother is my godmother and it was at his parents' wedding that I first met Tania. It was an interesting link – coming a full circle with me marrying Tania and now bumping into Alex many years later in West Africa. He had been accepted into my alma mater, Durham University, and was spending a gap year working for the United Nations. He was staying with British expats Nick and Kimberly Gardner and, as he had already been in Freetown for a month, offered to show me around. This was most welcome as my vehicle was effectively impounded.

Alex was a great companion. He was not only high-spirited, but also adventurous. After work he would meet me at the IMATT gate on his motorbike. I would get on another bike and we would buzz around the city, shopping and going to bars, doing things that young men do – although those days were long gone for me.

One memorable afternoon we booked a tour and set off for the east side of the town on Kroo Bay with a guide. There was a lot to see and the area had a fascinating, albeit often tragic, past.

First stop was Hill Station, a collection of crumbling wooden bungalows built at the top of an escarpment. In the early 1900s it had been an exclusive resort for British colonial administrators, built on stilts for cooler air to pass through and provide some respite from mosquitoes. Queen Elizabeth stayed there when she visited the country in 1961 and although it's now badly rundown, it still has a certain charm.

We then went down the hill to St John's Maroon church, one of the oldest buildings in the country, constructed by Jamaican ex-slaves who were settled in the area in 1800. Next was the Cotton Tree, a giant kapok tree that was one of the city's most iconic symbols. This was where a group of formerly enslaved African Americans, who had gained their freedom by fighting for the British during the American Revolutionary War, first settled when they arrived in Sierra Leone on 11 March 1792. Sadly, the 230-foot kapok was brought down in a storm on 24 May 2023. A new monument containing remnants of the magnificent tree is to be built on the site.

Our guide then took us to the Connaught hospital, the country's principal referral hospital, opened in 1912 by the Duke of Connaught, Prince Arthur. A hospital may not be much of a tourist attraction, but on one rather weather-beaten gate was a plaque that simply states, 'In memory of the 150,000 Africans liberated by the West Africa Squadron, 1808 – 1860'. That certainly gave pause for thought. The West Africa Squadron was a fleet of Royal Navy warships based in Freetown that relentlessly patrolled the coastline, boarding slave ships at gunpoint and freeing the desperate human cargo chained in the hulls. Seventeen thousand sailors lost their lives during this period – one for every nine freed slaves. Most of the liberated slaves arriving in Sierra Leone came from a range of African countries as well as North America and the Caribbean, eventually forming a distinct ethnic group, the Krio, with their unique language and cultural forms. As a military man, I found this history fascinating and a poignant reminder in these revisionist times that sometimes might is right.

Strangely enough, soon afterwards I had my first and only personal experience of aggression in Africa. I was staying for a few days with Martin Bamin, a great bloke and former British soldier, who lived opposite a hotel called The Hub. It's a central meeting point and on most evenings I walked over for a coke or a beer. On one occasion a gate guard angrily refused to let me in for no reason at all. At first I assumed it was because the president or someone important was visiting, but the guard belligerently told me in no uncertain terms to scarper. I told him I regularly visited the hotel, but it made no difference. It was pretty obvious that he had taken a dislike to me, either for my rather scruffy appearance (difficult to comb your hair when you have Parkinson's), or perhaps my skin colour. It was my first experience of this, as even when my Mauritanian 'friend' Omaar had ripped me off, it had all been rather good-natured.

Not this time. The gate guard was literally bristling with hostility – and although minor in the extreme, it did give me some small indication of how millions of black people must have felt when they were denied entry into establishments during the discriminatory days of England or, even worse, apartheid South Africa. Nothing came of it, of course, as I was not going to challenge a fit, athletic young man in my debilitated state, but it was ironic that it happened in a country where a significant number of people have slave forebears, making it perhaps easier to understand. In any event, I went to the bar again later and another gate guard let me in with a smile.

Although Covid was spreading like wildfire in the UK, with draconian lockdowns now in force, there were still no recorded cases in Sierra Leone. Consequently, I was pretty blasé about everything, although I knew I would soon have to make a decision on whether to continue the journey or go home. Luckily, a British military officer with IMATT, Matt Palmer and his wife Jane, invited me to stay with them in their very comfortable house, so my short-term accommodation was secure.

As far as I was concerned, I had four options; carry on motoring all the way to South Africa; return to the Sahara and live in the desert for a while; wait out the pandemic in Sierra Leone; catch a boat home – the only way I could get the wagon back to the UK. The more I thought about it, the keener I was to keep heading south to the tip of the continent. What did I have to lose? New adventures and exploring new countries? Yes, please.

So that was it. I would continue to South Africa.

No sooner had I made up my mind than the British high commission announced they were evacuating all non-essential staff back to the UK. This did not include me as I was a civilian, but it did include Matt and Jane Palmer, who were given three days to pack up. It also meant I had to find somewhere else to stay.

At that point, Martin Travers came to my rescue. A former officer, he had left the Army and was now working as an advisor to the mayor of Freetown, a job paid for by the Tony Blair Foundation. I had met Martin and his wife Jenny once or twice and on the strength of those chance meetings they offered me a room in their house and a place to park the wagon. They could not have been more kind and for the next three weeks I stayed with them. There was still no lockdown or curfew in Freetown, so life was pleasant enough and I spent a lot of time on the capital's renowned beaches. Sierra Leone was no stranger to pandemics, with fairly regular outbreaks of Ebola and residents were used to social distancing when necessary. There were plenty of handwashing stations.

Soon afterwards, all African borders started closing and it seemed I had little option but to stay where I was until the pandemic ended. Imagine my surprise when I was given the option to buy a ticket on one of the last commercial flights out of the country. Initially, I wasn't keen, but friends provided some convincing evidence that it was in my best interests to get out while I could. I went to the Air France office the next morning and I was able to book a ticket on a flight the following week. Alex was also scheduled to leave that day.

Just as I finished packing everything up and was ready to go, I got an urgent message from Air France. The flight had been cancelled. I was stuck again, with seemingly no way out. The plan now was simply to stay with Martin and Jenny until the pandemic blew over. There was nothing else I could do and it was my incredible good fortune to have linked up with such generous people, otherwise I would have been in a real jam.

A couple of days later, a nurse contacted me and said there was a flight to Brussels organised by the European Union that had a seat available. Although the UK was no longer a member of the EU, they were prepared to make exceptions for vulnerable Brits. The nurse was adamant that I leave. 'If the pandemic gets out of control, Freetown is not the place to be. If you get ill there will be no one to look after you and it'll be serious.'

I somewhat reluctantly agreed and a few days later was instructed to go to the German embassy to pick up a ticket and be ready to fly within forty-eight hours. It was a sad moment saying goodbye to Martin and Jenny. Over a short period they had become exceptionally good friends. They said I could leave the wagon and I quickly gave their driver Solomon instructions on how to look after the vehicle.

Then Sierra Leone introduced their first lockdown. Not only that, it would come into force at midnight the day before

I was due to fly out. No one could travel anywhere without written government permission. This meant that I had to get two permits, as a trip to Lungi airport also involved a forty-minute water taxi ride across the bay. I needed authorisation to get driven to the docks, as well as to board the boat.

The EU plane arrived empty and as there were no passengers disembarking, it was a quick turn around and we were soon in the air. I think I was the only Brit on board.

Eight hours later I landed in Brussels, expecting a short hiatus and confident I'd be back in Sierra Leone three months later. At the most.

It was instead two years.

23

Back Home

It was surreal boarding the Eurostar train in Brussels to find I was almost the only passenger. St Pancras station in London was equally deserted, but my sister Tina had hired a driver to take me to my mother's house in Wiltshire, where I picked up a car that she wasn't using to travel to Tania in Scotland.

I didn't get close enough to speak to my mother – one thing we did know about Covid at that point was that elderly people were particularly vulnerable – and was only able to wave at her through the window as I drove off.

Tania had moved house while I was in Africa and was now renting a smallish place in the countryside outside Perth. Our two children were also there, working from home during lockdown and although one barely dares admit it, we had a wonderful time walking Walter, our new labrador, and cycling in perfect weather. Even the winter was memorable, with plenty of snow and with few people in the countryside, Tania and Millie regularly skied in the Grampian Mountains on our doorstep. It had been quite a while since the four of us had been under the same roof at the same time, so lockdown was good to us.

However, I was still determined to continue the odyssey and spent countless hours planning and dreaming about the second half of the journey. Despite the fact that thousands more people in the UK had Covid than did in Sierra Leone, I now accepted that coming home was the right thing to do. Not only had I been running low on Parkinson's pills in Africa, but as everyone had warned, it would have been serious if I had fallen ill there. In retrospect, circumstances proved that I was lucky to get out when I did. If I had pushed on, I would almost certainly have found myself stranded in either Guinea or Liberia with all borders shut and very limited opportunities to get medication.

But even so, it was difficult getting used to not having the wagon and all my stuff a mere arm's reach away. I missed the vast desert expanses, the acacias of the Sahel, the rolling savannahs and wild Atlantic beaches. Indeed, at times I didn't know what to do with myself without having an engine to tinker with or bolts to tighten. But thanks to Miriam in Senegal, I had a gazillion Senegalese music tracks to sort through while I edited my photographs. Even though I was thousands of miles away in central Scotland, I was in Africa in spirit.

Nothing was set in stone at that stage but my rough plan was to return to Sierra Leone and, as soon as Africa's land borders opened, I would continue south-east to Liberia and the Ivory Coast into Ghana, from where I would try and catch a ferry to Angola. That meant I would cut out a number of difficult border crossings by avoiding Nigeria, Cameroon, Gabon and both Congos. Once in southern Angola the roads would get better, the weather more benign and the environment less harsh. It might be a bit of a copout taking a boat, which would undermine the overland ethos of the odyssey, but I was not trying to prove anything to anyone.

With enforced isolation, it was also now time to take stock of my health. Alarmingly, despite being back home on full medication and eating regular nutritious meals, my Parkinson's was getting worse. This was strange, as with no real stress to deal with, not to mention no mosquitoes or extreme heat, I should've actually felt better. Yet I found myself moving slower than I had ever before and my already precarious balance was even more shaky. The inexorable march of Parkinson's was significantly more measurable and my latest frustration was trying to press keys on a mobile phone or iPad. No matter how carefully I aimed, I nearly always hit the wrong one.

But I was beginning to discover that the worst thing about Parkinson's is not the physical limitations. Grim as they are, that's the boring side. Far more pernicious is the effect the disease has on one's desire to be with other people and to enjoy life. It destroys that basic community need we all have, undermining one's confidence to the point of giving up. I started to think of myself as being unworthy of people's attention and care. The disease was destroying my self-esteem and that's what I hated most about it. Knowing that tomorrow will be worse than today is depressing beyond belief.

I often describe Parkinson's this way: if by some quirk of timing I found myself in the middle of the road with a bus coming fast at me, I would certainly try to get out of the way however fast my shuffling would let me. But frankly I wouldn't mind if it hit me. We are all going to die one day and while there are key family milestones I would like to be around for, there are greater Parkinson's-imposed milestones I would not mind avoiding!

I suffer from a particular type of Parkinson's where I move very slowly. I don't shake uncontrollably like many other sufferers and tend to be motionless when sitting. As a result, people think I'm not interested in what they're saying or doing, which is not the case at all. I just can't express anything through body language. In fact, I can sometimes barely move without my routine dosage of up to twelve pills a day.

Consequently, I am not surprised when people either ignore or speak to me only out of a sense of duty. I believe I'm bad company and feel sorry for anyone finding themselves sitting next to me at a dinner party where I'm not only scruffy and my eating and drinking techniques are unattractive, but I'm slow to join in conversations – let alone provide witty entertainment for my unlucky neighbour.

To add to the sense of unworthiness, when people waiting in a queue see someone like me stumbling and fumbling to insert a cash card or get cash out of their wallets, they get frustrated and impatient and I do not blame them. They don't know that underneath that bumbling exterior is an ordinary person, wrestling day and night with this dreadful affliction. For most of us sufferers, we're still the same people underneath.

Parkinson's is not only incurable, it's also degenerative and the drugs merely manage the decline rather than turn it around. And there was no doubt that my deterioration was speeding up. Yet being aware of this didn't mean I had to stop trying – if anything, it strengthened my resolve. I now wanted to continue the odyssey more than anything else, even though I couldn't do up my buttons, comb my hair or shave. I was increasingly aware that the second stage of the journey was going to be even more difficult, but a peculiar tenacity took hold. I knew what I had to do and added to this stubbornness was now the hope that my example might inspire others. Perhaps they would look at me and say, 'If that old git can do it, anyone can.'

Although keen as mustard to continue, I was still little more than a helpless bystander in a world spinning out of control. My initial assumption that the pandemic would be over in three months proved to be laughably wrong. After a year had passed I'd reached the stage where I wondered if we would ever emerge from lockdowns. I began to doubt if I would ever get back to my wagon in Africa.

But I never gave up hope.

In early 2021, we moved out of our house in Scotland to Leigh, about five miles from Sherborne where the odyssey had started in November 2019. I always wanted to return to Dorset, as although Scotland is beautiful and I spent seven good years on and off working there, it was not home.

Lockdown restrictions gradually started to ease and I drove to Bristol to meet up with Peter Robinson, an old university friend, for lunch. As fate would have it, his daughter was there and she introduced me to her boyfriend, Rob Hayward.

Rob is the creative director and co-founder of the Bristol-based film company Newfruit Productions, which specialises in making motivational corporate videos. We got chatting and when I told him about the African odyssey and Parkinson's, he immediately asked if I had any film of the voyage.

'Right here,' I said, and handed him my phone.

I had taken a lot of photos and video clips for my Polarsteps blog and Rob had a look at that as well as some great footage David Attenburrow had shot in the Sahara. Some of my stuff was a little amateurish but Rob seemed genuinely blown away by the overall story. In turn, I could sense that he had a passion for great filmmaking.

During our conversation we both had a lightbulb moment in seeing the potential to make a documentary of the voyage, but now we remember the crux of the discussion differently. I recall him saying he wanted to do it, but he remembers me asking him to do so. No one is sure who initiated the project, but the end result was that both of us wanted to shoot a film when Africa's borders reopened.

This added a new focus to my mission. After meeting Rob, there was a sudden surge of interest in what I was doing. It was both humbling as well as a huge shot in the arm to continue.

In fact, it was life-changing.

24

Change of Focus

Top priority now was to raise funds. Shooting a full-length, high-quality documentary costs a lot of money and even though Rob and I would be unpaid, we still needed to buy equipment and cover production and editing costs.

The easiest and probably most effective way to finance this would be to create a page on a crowdfunding website. I was warned that most appeals fail, but we had little choice.

First, we needed to make a short promotional video to attract donors and to do this we used a barn owned by Andrew Spink in Dorset as a backdrop where I outlined the aim of the odyssey. I stressed that although it was an ambitious project, I was already halfway through the journey and my track record showed I'd never baulked at anything just because it was difficult.

Rob shot the bulk of the film on a cold winter's day and the barn was freezing, so I looked more miserable than I was. It took two afternoons to complete, and for the first time I witnessed the extraordinary attention to detail required to make a good film into an excellent film. It was then that I appreciated how lucky I was to have met up by chance with a young chap who wanted to make a film about a knackered old man realising his dream.

We posted the video on Indiegogo.com, one of the first sites to offer crowdfunding, as well as the networking site LinkedIn.

Most LinkedIn users are at the senior end of their profession and many would have elderly parents, some of whom might be affected by Parkinson's. Rob and I decided it was a perfect target market, as those who knew something about Parkinson's would be supportive, while those who didn't would hopefully be interested in my story.

It worked. Beyond all expectations. The film was seen by thousands and it struck a chord. One remark I particularly remember was from a three-star general who told me he was reduced to tears and could not watch it through to the end. Rob and I had many similar comments from other viewers and their generosity was staggering. For example, a person I'd never heard of – and who probably had never heard of me before seeing the film – instantly donated a thousand pounds. I personally phoned to thank him.

Most people of means I knew had already donated, but I approached them again, thanking them for their prior generosity but asking if this time they wouldn't mind acting on my behalf and contacting anyone else they knew who might be prepared to assist. Although donations were coming in, what we really needed was, say, five people to donate ten thousand pounds each and we would reach our goal. The idea was to get a small number of big hitters, rather than the other way around.

Then I got a call from an old friend, Gil Baldwin, the non-executive chairman of the health plan provider Simplyhealth. Gil is an extremely loyal friend and had supported me and Fiona Tanner when we ran marathons to raise funds for Parkinson's more than a decade ago. He said he would speak to his board and soon afterwards Rob and I hit our target.

We could now make the film.

In the promotional clip Rob had inserted some rather harrowing footage provided by Omotola Thomas's charity Parkinson's Africa, which proved to be very effective. The work Omotola has done is staggering. To have the energy and drive to get such a huge project off the ground when stricken by one

153

of the most debilitating illnesses as well as being the mother of two young children simply beggars belief. She now lives in Surrey with her family and was keen to make it clear that it's not all bad news for those afflicted with Parkinson's in Africa. There are a lot of people doing tremendous work, not to mention making great strides in dispelling the unfortunate stigmatisation in some quarters that Parkinson's is a curse rather than a disease. She was the first to admit that the harsh reality many medical officers on the continent face is that there are scores of other even more pressing problems – malaria and Ebola to name just two. Also, with life expectancy anyway being below fifty-eight years in many African countries, a significant number die before contracting Parkinson's, which usually affects people over sixty. However, life expectancy is increasing with better living standards and by 2040 it is estimated that a quarter of all Parkinson's sufferers will be in Africa. Some may believe that Parkinson's is not a big deal when viewed in a wider perspective, but that's a very short-sighted approach.

I initially had been introduced to Omotola by Helen Matthews before leaving on my odyssey in 2019. At that meeting I had made vague promises that I would try and visit Parkinson's sufferers and see specialists treating the disease, which I failed to do in Morocco and Mauritania. I didn't get the correct contacts in advance, so found it difficult to organise media and visits to treatment centres while on the move. As a result, my role as a Parkinson's ambassador was not all-consuming.

This time it would be different. I would use Omotola's contacts as well as various British embassies and their media links to meet as many of those at the coalface of the Parkinson's struggle as possible. By making a movie, I had a lot more gravitas, so to speak. People would take me far more seriously as I was no longer just a random bloke with a logo on the side of his van.

The aim of the journey would now be far more focused. The message was one of hope; that Parkinson's can be beaten if not cured and need not ruin one's life. Also, this time around, with

Omotola's and official Foreign Office help, I had a network of influential contacts in advance, including in the media, to get the message across. And, of course, I would be banging on about the availability and exorbitant expense of medication, taking it way out of reach of the vast majority of sufferers. That was something close to my heart, as it was one aspect I had experienced personally on the first half of the journey.

In short, I hoped that my odyssey would contribute in some small way to easing the burden and finding a cure for this illness – not necessarily for me or my generation as I fear that ship has sailed. Instead, it would be for those who come after.

There were now encouraging signs that Covid travel restrictions would be lifted and I wanted to start getting provisions and vital spare vehicle parts shipped out to Sierra Leone. Some of this was guesswork, as it was difficult to know exactly what I would need without having the wagon nearby to inspect everything. However, one thing I did know was that the next stage of the voyage would be through some of the worst, muddiest and most treacherous roads in Africa. It would be far trickier than the first section, and I found myself becoming increasingly daunted. I had to deliver, no matter how rapidly my Parkinson's was deteriorating. It was no longer just me leisurely heading south any more as Rob and I had raised a lot of money and promised results for our backers.

But even in my darkest moments, never once did I contemplate not finishing the journey. I knew I would not get this chance again.

At last, in February 2022, travel restrictions were lifted. It had been two long years, and once everything was back on track, my misgivings vanished. I was now champing at the bit to get back to Africa.

This time I had added focus. As well as a movie to make.

25

Back to Africa

Covid restrictions might have been eased, but lingering problems remained. Not least was the fact that anyone travelling to Sierra Leone had to have a medical certificate stating they were Covid-free.

These certificates were valid for three days and as I was flying out on Monday at 5 a.m., I had to get Covid clearance on the Saturday at significant expense. I emailed this through to the Sierra Leone embassy, acknowledgment only arriving at 2 a.m. on Monday, a mere hour before I was scheduled to check in. Fortunately, I had anticipated this and stayed at a Heathrow airport hotel, just managing to get on board the flight in time, but it was a close call. As mentioned, with Parkinson's, extreme anxiety is exponentially triggered by even mild stress and this was no exception. I couldn't even get the ticket out of my pocket and an airline assistant had to sort out all my paperwork.

Landing in Sierra Leone nine hours later was vastly different from my arrival two years previously, when I spent forty-eight hours at the border post trying to get clearance for my right-hand drive van. This time I had VIP treatment, being greeted by a fixer from the British high commission. He whisked me through customs and onto a water taxi across the bay to Freetown, where I met up with Martin and Jenny Travers.

I would be staying with them once again while I prepared the wagon for the next stage, which included making sure I had adequate provisions as the next country I would be visiting, Liberia, is one of the most destitute on the continent.

I also appeared on local TV, something I now planned to do in every country, hammering home the message of my journey. I found that journalists were generally keen to interview me. What got me through the media door, so to speak, was the news angle, 'Who's this madman driving all this way across Africa?' This then moved to, 'Who is this madman driving all this way with Parkinson's?' And, finally, 'What is Parkinson's?' Within no time we would be talking about Parkinson's itself, which was the core issue.

What helped more than anything else was that the new British high commissioner, Lisa Chesney, was genuinely interested in my story. The previous assistant defence attaché, John Harper, had also been excellent when I was first in the country (it's not just me saying that; he was awarded a MBE for his work) but Lisa took it even further, instructing her press department to use their clout with the media. From that moment on I knew my journey had taken on far more significance than I ever thought possible. A greater number of influential people knew about what I was doing. To my surprise there was even some admiration that I'd got as far as I had before the Covid outbreak.

Consequently, I did a lot of interviews, and high commission staff often accompanied me in case I had issues such as fatigue or anxiety while live on national TV. They were very conscious that, despite everything, the bottom line was that I had advanced Parkinson's.

Fortunately, all press interviews went well, and I believe I gave a decent account of myself. I'd had a fair amount of prior experience in dealing with the press – Princess Anne's trip to Belize being a case in point – but it was a first for most African journalists to find themselves interviewing a Parkinson's sufferer. There is little doubt that being on TV brought the issue of what Parkinson's actually is – a disease not a stigma – into many Sierra Leoneans' living rooms.

I had the pleasure as well of stumbling across some members of my old regiment. It happened completely by chance – I was sitting at a beach restaurant minding my own business when several young Brits appeared. They immediately caught my attention, as although they wore civilian clothes, to the trained eye they were obviously soldiers. Granted, they were carrying army-style rucksacks and wearing tactical watches, but I can recognise a soldier from a mile away.

We got chatting and to my delight, they told me they were from the Queen's Dragoon Guards. My surprise at hearing that was nothing compared to theirs at meeting a former colonel dressed in a purple polo shirt, faded black swimming trunks and barefoot on a sun-drenched beach in West Africa. Although they didn't know me personally, they knew who I was. Thinking back on my past exploits with the QDG – from the Cold War frontline to the Teleki expedition – it was gratifying to know that the Army still sent soldiers to remote corners to help other countries and have an epic adventure along the way.

In fact, Sierra Leone has a strong military attachment to the UK, as it was thanks to British soldiers that the rebel forces of the Revolutionary United Front (RUF) were defeated during the civil war that raged from 1992–2002. Fifty thousand civilians were killed in that conflict, and it was brutal beyond description. RUF fighters, usually drugged to their eyeballs, offered their captives 'short or long sleeve' options. A short sleeve was amputation above the elbow; a long sleeve at the wrist. Not being infantry, the QDG did not fight in that war but even so, I was told by my new friends that my old regiment routinely sent a small number of troops to help train the Sierra Leonean forces.

While waiting for my visa to Liberia to be approved, Martin Travers's tour of duty ended and he would be leaving Freetown to take up a post elsewhere. As a result, I had to relocate to a bed-and-breakfast about a mile down the road. It was rough and ready with no air conditioning, food or fridge, just water and a fan, but I supposed as that was how I was going to be living when on the road, I might as well get used to it.

However, the biggest problem was that I had to move the van from Martin's former house, which I could not do without Department of Transport permission. After all the hassles last time, I at least now knew what had to be done and with Martin's driver Solomon's help, banged on various doors and got through to the right people fairly quickly. The official in charge would only give me permission to drive the van out of the country and said I'd have three days to do so once the permit was granted. He consequently suggested I get the permit stamped at the last moment to give me as much time to reach a border as possible. But this meant I could not move the wagon off Martin's premises. Well, not legally. So we did the only thing possible – sneaking it down the road to my new accommodation at midnight when, fortunately, no police were around. We also got it serviced that way, parking it at a garage in the early morning so the mechanics could work on it during the day, then clandestinely driving it back after dark.

Finally, the border with Liberia opened and Rob Hayward flew out to film me preparing for the next stage and joined me on the drive to Liberia. Although some of the money raised through crowdfunding went to buying equipment and teaching me better filming techniques, we also had designated funds for Rob to fly out at various stages of the journey. We knew I would not be able to film it all myself and, as it happened, I needed him to come out for longer than we had initially budgeted.

I held a farewell party at a delightful restaurant called Mango Peak, where we invited the press, high commission staff as well as anyone who had helped us in some way and it was a great send off. I was interviewed by TV, again highlighting the plight of Parkinson's victims and then we were on the road.

Not for long. A few hours later, just before Bo, the second city of Sierra Leone, a nastier pothole than usual bent two wheel rims. The only solution was to bash them back into shape, replace the most damaged one with a spare and take it to a garage in Bo to get repaired. We then camped the next night at Tiwai Island, a small nature reserve that was reputed to be a good place to view primates. We didn't see any.

The following morning, we arrived at the Liberian border.

26

Liberia

A huge Liberian who introduced himself as Edward met us at the border. He was about 6 feet 6 inches and built like an ox and we were extremely happy to see him. He was our fixer, who would get us through customs.

Edward worked for Henderson Risk Limited, an insurance company that does private security in Africa and whose CEO, Duncan Bullivant, had been my second-in-command in A Squadron during the Cold War era. Duncan had heard of my journey and said his company would help pave the way in some of the potentially more difficult countries. The magnanimity of that assistance, particularly in Liberia and Nigeria, was profound as unfortunately corruption is rife at the various border posts. Edward was there to see corruption didn't affect us at the Liberian crossing and with his imposing presence it didn't.

Our first stop was Robertsport, about ten miles from the border and named after Joseph Jenkins Roberts, Liberia's first president. It's a rather charming village and one of the country's best tourist venues, or so I'm told, as there were only four foreigners there when we arrived. However, it's still suffering from the ravages of the two civil wars and many of the rather pleasant, plantation-style houses are riddled with bullet pockmarks. It's mostly a fishing village, but is also getting a reputation as a surfing resort as there are five different point breaks along a spectacular beach lined with coconut and mango trees. Americans coming to the area after the 2003 peace treaty taught the locals how to surf and Robertsport beach boys have continued the tradition.

Interestingly, a tree growing where Joseph Roberts first landed in Liberia after sailing from America in 1829 still stands. The port was also an Allied submarine base during the Second World War.

We stayed for two and a half days, enjoying being by the sea, while Rob did some pieces to camera with waves breaking in the background. Fortuitously, a Swedish couple, Theresa and Andreas, were at the same guesthouse and, as they were leaving for Monrovia at the same time, offered to show us the easiest route into the teeming city. This was good news as it had just started raining, an ominous forewarning that it would soon be West Africa's monsoon season where rainfall can exceed 40 inches.

Rob was flying out to England the next day and I dropped him off at a hotel within easy striking distance of Roberts International airport, then followed Andreas into Monrovia. It's impossible to say much positive about the capital city, particularly as the entrance consists of slums and squatter markets spilling into the potholed road. Consequently, it was extremely useful to be following someone with local knowledge.

I then met up with Henry Joynson and Ian Currie, who also worked for Henderson Risk. I would be staying with them for the next two weeks. Henry is an old army friend and a true adventurer. He has hundreds of medals for every type of military operation you can imagine and reminds me of the swashbuckling buccaneers of yesteryear. It was great to see him again, as well as Ian, a kindred spirit with a Royal Navy pedigree. I could not have asked for better company in a less secure country.

I wanted to do some press interviews and Andreas and Theresa invited me to meet the Swedish ambassador. His office was on the floor above the British embassy and after exchanging formalities, I visited the British ambassador, Neil Bradley. He was really helpful and his staff provided media contacts and also arranged for me to meet Liberia's impressive chief medical officer, Dr Francis Kateh.

Thanks to the ambassador, the press was interested in my story and one of my first interviews was a phone-in with a radio station. I got quite a surprise when a high-ranking politician, whose mother had recently died with Parkinson's, personally rang in to say he would do more to foster awareness of the disease with the chief medical officer. I'm not sure what came of that – or even that I got the gist of the conversation right – as although the official language of Liberia is English, it has a particular Caribbean lilt that is difficult to grasp at first. However, I knew that the phone-in had been a success, as at least two people approached me on separate occasions some days later when they saw my van's logo, saying they had heard me on the radio and wanted to know what they could do to help. It was extremely gratifying.

A day later, I quietly gatecrashed a cocktail party at the French embassy to mark the opening of an Alliance Française language centre, as I hoped to meet someone interesting there. I certainly did – her name was Sadia and she had worked at the Liberian embassy in Germany. She told me her uncle, Patrick Massaquoi, had Parkinson's and wanted me to speak to him. I agreed enthusiastically as he would be the first person I had met in Africa who had the disease. He lived about thirty minutes' drive from Monrovia, and three days later Sadia took me to her uncle's humble home, where he stayed with his wife and son.

Patrick was probably in his mid-sixties and, with no drugs, was a quivering wreck, existing day-to-day in his own sad world. He could barely talk or move, but the look on his face articulated his story more than any words could. He was having a horrible time. His son, who selflessly looked after him, was brilliant, showing what true caring was all about.

I explained I had Parkinson's as well and outlined what I was trying to do in telling the rest of the world about people like him and me. I said he was not alone and I would do my best to highlight the need to produce drugs more cheaply while we waited for a cure, which might not be in our lifetime. With all Parkinson's-afflicted people that I meet, I am very careful to speak generally and not to be specific in any individual cases. I simply can't make promises that I might not be able to keep.

I left feeling weak and despondent. The meeting was a precursor of what awaited me with the condition and, more importantly, a graphic snapshot of what people with Parkinson's in Africa face every day. It was a stark reminder of exactly what this trip was all about.

There was not much to do in Liberia as the damage is all pervasive, both physically and mentally, from the two brutal civil wars lasting from 1989 to 2003. Quarter of a million people died in the conflicts. Understandably, the long-suffering nation is extremely downbeat and the dominant obsession of many young people seems to be to make enough money to leave for America, legally or otherwise.

They say a picture tells a thousand words and the best view – and sadly also a metaphor – of Monrovia is from the top of the Ducor Hotel, West Africa's first five-star resort. The building sits on the highest point of the city overlooking the Atlantic Ocean, the Saint Paul River estuary and West Point, the capital's most densely populated slum district.

Built in 1960, the Ducor boasted 106 luxury rooms on eight stories and was the envy of the rest of Africa. Guests included global celebrities, presidents and business moguls. Idi Amin, the tyrant who expelled all Indians from Uganda in 1972, is said to have swum in the hotel pool while carrying his firearm, although I doubt that even in its heyday the hotel would have bragged about that.

During the war, it was looted to the bone and squatters moved in en masse. Today it is a skeletal shell of its former glory and, despite attempts at renovation, the once grand establishment remains a mute testimony to a shattered society.

The civil war is stuff of bizarre legends, not least being the story of General Butt Naked. The self-appointed general, so-called due to his penchant for going into battle without a stitch of clothing, was accused of child sacrifice and cannibalism. In the country's Truth and Reconciliation Commission held after the civil war, General Butt Naked admitted that his soldiers – the Naked Base Commandos – had killed up to twenty thousand civilians.

However, Africa being Africa, a continent where incredible forgiveness often exceeds violence, the muscle-bound and well-endowed General Butt Naked – whose real name is Joshua Milton Blahyi – is now a preacher in Monrovia. He claims to have seen the error of his ways and has undergone a Damascene conversion to Christianity.

I already had my visa for the Ivory Coast, my next destination, but while in Liberia also got visas for Togo and Benin as well. I set off for the border with one of Henderson's drivers provided by Ian, who was worried about security in the eastern part of the country.

The road heading for the Ivory Coast was a newly built Chinese road which, after several hours, surprisingly petered out to a basic mud track with low-hanging branches scraping the windscreen. It took us an hour to cover about five miles, and I could hardly believe we were on the right road. Eventually, the mud tracks opened up into a village, where a piece of string was strung across the road.

This was the border.

The Liberian customs officials checked everything was in order and let me through. No doubt the presence of my Liberian driver helped matters and, with his job done, he caught a taxi back to Monrovia.

I drove over a bridge only to find the other side chained up. As I was wondering what to do next, a guard emerged from a building and opened a padlock, releasing the chains.

I was now in the Ivory Coast. Or, as it is perhaps better known, Côte d'Ivoire.

27

Ivory Coast

As the only traveller at the border post, I expected to be whisked through fast. It didn't take long to be disabused of that notion. Even though I had a newly stamped visa, a valid passport and all my vehicle documentation was in order, I still had to go through three separate processes: immigration, customs and police. All asked the same questions and all wanted to see more or less the same documents. But that wasn't the only inconvenience. I had to visit each department in the right sequence; if I went to the police before customs, I would have to repeat the entire process. Even worse, the three departments don't seem to talk to one another, so I was not sure of the correct pecking order.

It eventually took me an hour and a half to do all this correctly, so I hate to imagine what it would have been like if there had been a queue. But even getting everything in the right order was no guarantee of success. In this case, the only person authorised to sign my police clearance form was not present. Feeling my stress levels soaring alarmingly, I resigned myself to spending a frustrating night at the border.

Suddenly, I was given a break. The 'missing' policeman was in Danané, a town about twenty miles east and I would be allowed to find him. His phone number was scribbled down, and I was on my way. I had planned to stop in Danané anyway as I needed to draw cash. As usual, I arrived in the fairly large town at sunset and, doubting that the immigration policeman I needed to phone would still be on duty, I decided to find a hotel. It was pouring with rain, reminding me that the monsoon forerunners were now travelling faster than I was.

Instead of starting early the next day to overtake the rain, I had to get my customs clearance signed. I phoned the policeman and was told to come to his office, but on arrival found he was missing in action once again. Instead, several of his officious colleagues started giving me a rough time, telling me to go back to the border. I nodded and hurriedly left. There was no way I was going to go through that rigmarole again and I decided to carry on travelling inland and take my chances. I had wasted enough time trying to do the right thing in any event.

Leaving Danané, I turned onto the main road to Yamoussoukro and the massive Basilica of Our Lady of Peace, which is even bigger than St Peter's in the Vatican and was high on my African bucket list. While passing through Dualla about ninety miles west of Yamoussoukro, I decided on the spur of the moment to stop for the night and checked into a hotel. No big deal – it was just one of those downbeat Parkinson's days that were becoming increasingly common and I was feeling knackered.

At the hotel I bumped into Christaline and Albéric de Colnet, a French couple who worked in Abidjan and had been hiking in the spectacular surrounding hills with their two children. They invited me to join them for supper by the swimming pool and we got chatting about various topics, including Parkinson's. It was an interesting evening – not to mention extraordinarily fortuitous, as it later turned out.

The next morning, I set off for the basilica along a four-lane highway built, as was often the case elsewhere, by the Chinese. When approaching the outskirts of the city, the four lanes became six, which seemed excessive as at times I was the sole vehicle on the road. Parts of the city also seemed deserted, radiating a weird sense of urban isolation that I hadn't encountered anywhere else in West Africa. I was sort of expecting this. I had been told that Yamoussoukro was the administrative capital in name only and everything important – economically, culturally or socially – still happened in Abidjan. This was starkly evident and although there were wonderful government buildings and apartment blocks, very few people seemed to live or work in them.

The focal point, of course, is the 518-foot-tall basilica but, although it's magnificent, I was not sure if it was worth the long detour needed to reach it. I'm glad I did as it is globally renowned as being the largest Christian church in the world, covering 320,000 square feet and seating eighteen thousand worshippers with space for another 300,000 outside. It was consecrated by Pope John Paul II in 1990 amid political controversy, as some considered it to be a vanity project initiated by the president at the time, Félix Houphouët-Boigny. A stained-glass mural depicts the ex-president kneeling before Jesus, who is riding a blue donkey.

Félix Houphouët-Boigny, considered to be one of Africa's founding fathers, is still revered in many circles, and another Yamoussoukro landmark is the palace where he is buried. Although the palace itself is strictly off-limits to the public, the legendary crocodiles given to him as 'pets' by the former dictator of Mali, Moussa Traoré, are still a popular tourist attraction. These fearsome reptiles are kept in an artificial lake in front of the palace gates and there is no dispute that they have feasted on humans – not least being their former keeper, Dicko Toki, who looked after them for thirty-three years. Toki gave them pet names such as Capitaine and Chef de Cabinet and kept them in check using a blunt machete with which he would whack the creatures if they got too close. Unfortunately, according to witnesses, this failed on one occasion and he was dragged into the lake by Chef de Cabinet, never to be seen again.

The same fate awaited a mourner at President Houphouët-Boigny's funeral in 1993. Overcome with grief, the man, shouting, 'The president is dead, why should I live?' clambered over the fence and dived into the lake.

I wanted to get to Abidjan before nightfall and decided to give the famous crocodiles a miss. The road linking the main cities of Ivory Coast was the answer to my prayers: having endured potholes and roadworks for the last week I found myself on a first-class motorway cruising at normal speeds with not a squeak from the suspension. Relaxed and enjoying the drive and having sorted out my accommodation for the night, it seemed nothing could go wrong and I would even arrive in daylight. I was on a ladder up. Then, in the blink of an eye, I was sliding back down the longest snake ever – to square one. As I approached the city perimeter, I attempted to change down a gear and the engine suddenly started revving over the music. I even remember what was playing: 'Since You Been Gone' by Rainbow.

I tried to change again, to no avail. The gears wouldn't mesh and it seemed as if the clutch had collapsed. It was like putting my foot down on a sponge.

I freewheeled the van onto the hard shoulder, hoping – in fact, praying – that I hadn't destroyed the clutch. A key symptom of a burnt-out clutch is the pungent stink of scorched rubber/brake pad, but as one of the many problems with Parkinson's is an inability to smell, I couldn't tell.

To add to my woes, I had broken down in a shanty town and was soon surrounded by a crowd. On the face of it I was in deep water – incapable of moving, a menacing crowd gathering, no friends in Abidjan to call for help and the consequences of Parkinson's surging at the first hint of a stressful situation. Fortunately, the crowd seemed friendly and wanted to help, but their eagerness was overpowering. Within moments they had opened the bonnet and were tinkering with the engine while I looked underneath to see if clutch fluid was leaking or if the cable had snapped.

It was soon obvious that my roadside helpers knew even less than I did, but what was alarming was that the van's doors were now open, tools were strewn about, all my possessions were vulnerable and everything was spiralling out of control. I had no idea if anyone was pilfering my stuff as it was impossible to try and address the clutch problem as well as keep an eye on the pushing crowd.

I managed to shut the bonnet, get my tools inside and close the doors without trapping anyone inside, then suggested to my horde of helpers that they push me along the hard shoulder to a rough and ready petrol station which I could see in the distance. At that moment, the police arrived, telling me I couldn't stop on the side of the motorway and ordering me to move on.

I nodded in exasperation. 'That's exactly what I'm trying to do. But my clutch is broken.'

The police at least got the crowd under control, and I then asked if they could call a recovery truck. The policeman said he would and there was a garage not too far away.

Suddenly, I heard a voice call out in French, 'Hey, Guy, is everything all right?'

I looked up. It was Albéric and Christaline, whom I had met the night before at the Dualla hotel. Noticing the commotion, they had slowed down and by a stroke of unbelievable good luck, saw me surrounded by the jostling crowd.

'Umm... not really,' I replied.

'Let's get you out of here,' shouted Albéric above the noise.

Night was falling fast and he offered to tow the van to their apartment where I could spend the night, and we would contact the 'best garage in Abidjan' the next morning.

I was staggered by their spontaneous generosity – they had only met me twenty-four hours earlier. We hitched up a towline and a couple of hours later I was having dinner in their apartment overlooking the Ébrié Lagoon. They even moved their daughter out of her bedroom to make way for me to have a good night's sleep after a stressful day. While they didn't exactly save my life, they certainly saved the day.

The next morning, true to his word, Albéric rang Papi's Garage and a driver arrived to take the wagon away on a flatbed truck. When I visited the garage that afternoon, mechanics had already removed the front section to get to the clutch system and it looked as if it had been in a serious crash with even the headlights off. Papi told me the clutch had indeed burnt out and I obviously needed a new one. But even in the Ivory Coast, one of the more sophisticated countries in West Africa, that was far easier said than done. Equally serious was that – as I had suspected – both front shock absorbers were broken. They would also be difficult to source.

Albéric had said Papi's was the best garage in the country and I soon discovered this was no exaggeration. I got to know him and his son Johan well as I spent most days with them, scouring the internet trying to find suitable parts. Taking customer service to new heights, they also often took me for a drink at Che's Bar around the corner after work.

Eventually we gave up. We couldn't find a VW California clutch anywhere, and I had no option but to get one shipped out from the UK. To do so via a normal retail outlet would take a month or more and, with the monsoon season looming, it was time I simply did not have.

The fastest solution was for someone just to get on a passenger plane and smuggle a clutch into the country. Apparently, it's illegal for airline passengers to have motor spares in their luggage, so it was a big deal to ask someone to do that for me.

Once again, my friends came to my aid. On this occasion Hank Jansen, an old army buddy, volunteered to fly to Abidjan with the crucial package, while Rob Willis from Volkstrek not only found me the correct clutch, but drove it from Aberystwyth in Wales to Hank's home in Manchester. Hank wrapped each part of the clutch individually and stashed them as unobtrusively as he could in his hand luggage. There was a certain amount of apprehension passing the bag through the airport security X-ray machines, but somehow he got through.

Hank managed to slip through Ivory Coast customs without incident and we drove straight from the airport to deliver the brand new part to Papi. As Hank had come all this way, I was determined he was going to have a good holiday as a reward and rented an Airbnb within walking distance from the garage, not far from the beach.

Hank's arrival was a huge breath of fresh air. I had been having a miserable time worrying about the wagon and whether I would be stranded in the rains as I also had a strict deadline to meet Rob and Omotola in Ghana, my next stop. I could feel myself responding badly to all the stress. But it was hard to be downbeat with Hank around. Nothing gets him down and he has faced personal challenges that would defeat most of us. He was innately cheerful and Abidjan was a cosmopolitan city with lots of nightlife and restaurants. We ate and drank like kings and had a lot of laughs. Hank's father also had Parkinson's, so he knew what I was going through and what to do, or equally important, what not to do. Balancing the offer of help – when to give it and when not to – is an art that very few get right and he was extremely sensitive to my needs. I've known him for more than thirty years and could not have asked to have a better bloke around.

Within two days Papi's mechanics had fitted the clutch and there was more good news when a friend of Johan's found some VW shock absorbers while rummaging through a container of spares. They weren't the exact specification for the wagon, but would do the job. Or so we hoped. In any event, there was no option as they were the only ones available.

However, while fitting the shocks the mechanics discovered another problem – the prop shaft's retaining bracket had cracked due to the woeful roads, but Papi's ever-resourceful team welded it back into serviceable condition.

Papi charged nothing for the time his team had spent repairing the wagon and I only had to pay for the two shock absorbers. It was his astonishingly magnanimous gift to the

Parkinson's cause – generosity from the heart and in complete contrast to some of the tight-fisted multi-millionaires I later met on my travels.

To celebrate the wagon being on the road again, Papi took us out for drinks at Che's Bar. All of his mates were there and none of them would let me buy a round. They knew about my mission and, like Papi, this was their way of showing support.

Abidjan was certainly a city of interesting people and one of the most remarkable I met was Chloe Grant, an English expat who runs a WhatsApp group called West African Travellers. It's an invaluable sounding board for those either driving or backpacking through the area, providing a support system and sharing information on visas, border crossings, accommodation and fun things to do in each country. She's a veteran traveller herself, having previously worked for a West African airline, but now lives in Grand-Bassam, a UNESCO World Heritage Site just east of Abidjan with beautiful French colonial buildings. Nothing for her is too much trouble when it comes to helping others.

I spent an afternoon with her and her adopted son Patrick and although it was a social visit, it turned out to be incredibly useful. Chloe has excellent press contacts, something I needed badly as the British embassy in Abidjan was useless. In fact, the staff were worse than that; they were out-and-out unhelpful, refusing even to let me into their offices. All other British embassies had gone out of their way to support me, particularly with media liaison, so I resigned myself to temporarily winding down the Parkinson's awareness campaign while in the Ivory Coast.

Until I met Chloe. She put in touch with Thierry, a press fixer who – for a fee – would negotiate with the media on my behalf. What I hadn't known before was that you have to pay the Ivorian media to interview you, unlike the rest of the world where news value is the determining factor. If Chloe hadn't told me that, I would have got nowhere. As a result, Thierry got me interviews with a couple of newspapers, but even better, promised some TV coverage. Sure enough, just as I was about to leave for Ghana, he phoned to say that he had secured a slot on a TV programme called *C'midi*.

Initially, I thought it would be a low-key news channel, similar to others I had been on in Liberia and Sierra Leone.

I could not have been more wrong.

28

Meltdown

C'midi is a popular chat show on Ivorian daytime TV. It's screened before a live audience, and, as the name states, it's aired at midday.

The host was Caroline Dasylva, a household name in the Ivory Coast, although I didn't know that when I arrived at the studio at about 10 a.m. In fact, I was blissfully unaware that I was about to be a guest on the country's slickest flagship programme.

I was met by one of the production staff who asked for my phone to copy photos of the journey off it. I gave it to him, thinking it was a good idea, then forgot about it. Moments later I was whisked into a makeup room and that's when I had the first inkling of what I was in for. This was the big league and I suddenly got a little apprehensive. I was no stranger to being interviewed or dealing with the press, but it suddenly dawned on me that I would be talking about serious matters in a foreign language to a very large audience. Even the studio audience comprised at least two hundred people and my nerves increased when I saw the director priming them to clap, laugh and whoop with excitement.

The TV set was like a big aircraft hangar, smart and professional with a horseshoe-shaped table in the middle and Caroline Dasylva at the head. The guests – four Ivorian celebrities and me – flanked her, sitting on Parkinson's-unfriendly barstools that did little for my dodgy balance. But at least the discomfort kept me alert. And I had to be, as the discussion was not only in French, but delivered at a thousand words a minute. Although I got the gist of what was being said, I had to listen carefully for catchwords such as, 'Guy Deacon' (pronounced '*Gee Dee-kon*'), 'Parkinson's', 'voyage' – or even 'Volkswagen'. That would give me a clue when it was my turn to speak.

In my best Franglais, aided by a large studio screen showing background clips of the journey, I described my Parkinson's African odyssey and why I was doing it. Sometimes I was not exactly sure of the questions, so Caroline got whatever answer I thought suitable, whether she had asked for it or not. Whenever I used too many English words, she or the delightful guest next to me would assist with, 'What I think *Gee* is trying to say is…' My segment lasted an hour and by all accounts I didn't make too much of a fool of myself. Then, just before the end, Caroline said, 'I have something for you.'

She swivelled in her chair and a WhatsApp video clip flashed on the studio screen above. It was Tania and our children. That's why the producer had wanted my phone – not just for the photos, but to contact my wife. The message was simple and from the heart. 'Well done, Daddy. We're proud of you. We miss you. We love you.'

I stared silently at the screen for several moments, totally, utterly overwhelmed. It was the first time Millie and Wilfred had said anything like that. And to hear them saying it on national TV, albeit in a foreign country… well, I cried live on air. I'm not ashamed to admit it. Even today when I think about it, I shed tears. The audience loved it too.

As the show closed, I was physically and emotionally exhausted, not only from the concentration of speaking in a foreign language to a massive audience, but also the wonderful boost from my family. Caroline came over to thank me and the relief that I had held everything together under trying circumstances was enormous.

It was now about 1.30 p.m. and I decided I might as well head straight for the Ghana border, about 110 miles away. It would give me a running start as I had to be in Kumasi in three days' time to do more Parkinson's-related interviews with Omotola and Rob Hayward and his colleague Jack Chapman who were flying out to film that part of the trip.

I drove onto the urban motorway heading east, but somehow missed the turn-off for the road to the border via Grand-Bassam and got horribly lost. I was basically going round in circles and then realised that with the excitement of the TV show I had forgotten to take my midday Sinemet fix. I take two tablets three times a day, along with a dopamine enhancer. Without the drugs I go downhill quickly – which was exactly what was happening at that moment. I urgently needed to stop, take the pills and get my bearings, both physically and mentally.

Just ahead was a garage and I drove up to get a Coke to wash down the pills and eat a bar of chocolate. But, to my dismay, the garage didn't have a shop. There was a Carrefour supermarket, but it was on the other side of the highway and against the flow of traffic. It was easier to walk so, leaving the wagon on the garage forecourt, I managed to cross the busy highway without getting run over. I had to pass through a metal detector, similar to airport security. I put my personal effects in the plastic basket provided, taking stuff out of pockets with great difficulty thanks to my poor coordination and walked through the detector. But on collecting my belongings, I discovered my phone was missing.

Where's my phone? I started feeling all my pockets, looking around wildly. Within seconds I was in full-blown panic mode. My phone had everything on it: contacts, contactless payment, navigation apps – lots of essential stuff. I noticed a woman behind the desk looking at me, sensing my distress. 'My phone. It's been stolen from the basket,' I said.

She shook her head. 'That's not possible. Everything is there.'

'No, I'm telling you. I never go anywhere without my phone. I put the phone in and now it's gone.'

'Not possible,' she repeated.

I then lurched around to find someone who could speak English to communicate better and saw a white man. He might speak some English. He didn't, so I explained in French, aware that in my rising agitation I was becoming even more garbled. His eyes narrowed and he walked over to the woman I had just spoken to.

They conferred briefly, and I saw her vehemently shake her head.

He walked back to me. 'There was no phone.'

I was now intensely thirsty, suffering with dehydration that had been accelerated by excessive heat and soaring anxiety and I bought a disgusting fruit concentrate that I thought was Ribena. While trying to drink it, I slumped on the floor in a corner to try and stop the world from spinning.

A security guard came over. 'You can't stay here.'

'I'm doing no harm,' I replied, desperately trying to control my panic. Understandably, he thought I was ill – or perhaps drunk – and security staff manhandled me off the floor and half-dragged me to a back room. 'I've got to get my phone,' I said. 'Can't do without it.'

'We'll get you a doctor.'

'Also my car,' I said. 'It might be unlocked. All my worldly possessions are there. People will steal from it.'

'Where is it?' a woman asked.

'At the garage across the road. It's a VW campervan.'

She took my keys. 'I'll check if it's locked for you.'

A doctor arrived soon afterwards, checking my blood pressure and temperature but finding nothing too excessive, which was amazing considering the state I was in. He told me to rest for a while. I was so agitated I could only wait for ten minutes before I claimed to be better and the staff let me go.

Once outside, I saw an ambulance waiting. Surely it was not going to take me to hospital? My biggest fear was being admitted without doctors being aware of my medical history and in a strange city no one would know where I was, not even the useless embassy. It would also mean leaving the wagon – my home – unattended for some time.

Two big paramedics ran over, grabbed me and tried to force me into the ambulance. I resisted as strenuously as I could and it became a little like a Laurel and Hardy movie, with me repeatedly scrambling out of the ambulance as soon as they put me in. Eventually they held me down so I could not move.

'I've got Parkinson's,' I kept repeating. 'I've got to take some pills.'

While wrestling with the paramedics, a woman arrived and held up my keys. 'I've locked your car and here is your phone.' It was the Carrefour security guard. In my distressed state, I had forgotten about her. Not only had she checked the van was locked, but in doing so saw the phone on the seat. It had not been nicked after all!

My relief was infinite. 'Thank you. Thank you,' was all I could say.

She smiled and said, '*Ne rien.*' You are welcome. If anyone deserved employee of the year, she did.

The paramedics escorted me to the wagon, where I took my pills and phoned Chloe. She instantly sensed I was in a bad way when I passed my phone to one of the security guards to explain what had happened and where I was. She said she would send someone round to fetch me.

Not long afterwards, Thierry the press fixer arrived. Luckily, he had only just left the *C'midi* building and was able to get to me moments after Chloe's call. He immediately took control, telling the paramedics that I actually did have Parkinson's, as I had said, and he would look after me. He then booked someone to drive me and the wagon to Grand-Bassam.

When we reached Chloe's house, the emotional relief became physical. I rushed – or rather shuffled – to the loo as fast as I could, but not quite fast enough. I peed in my pants. In almost exactly three years, I had gone from being a proud cavalry colonel exchanging pleasantries with Prince William at Buckingham Palace to a quivering wreck who couldn't control his own bladder. I lay down and curled up into a ball in the shower.

Chloe, bless her, didn't mind.

29

Ghana

I took my pills, had a shower and spent the night at Chloe's. She was a lifesaver and I'm certainly not the first traveller she has helped out. Nor will I be the last.

The next morning, feeling a little more stable, I set off for Ghana, arriving at the Elubo border post about three hours later. I had been told that getting through land border crossings into Ghana was sometimes difficult as most tourists fly. I was prepared for a few hassles. Luckily, I knew a top-ranking Ghanaian army officer, Brigadier General Dan Frimpong, who was not only prepared to vouch for me, but personally knew the Ghanaian ambassador in the Ivory Coast. When I applied for a visa I took a letter from Dan stating that I was a good bloke and as a result I got special treatment – which also came in handy when a policeman stopped me and said I was not allowed to have a right-hand drive vehicle in Ghana. This was not true and I knew that only applied to Sierra Leone. When I showed him my 'credentials', his attitude did a quick U-turn and he waved me on my way.

Unfortunately, though, I was going the wrong way. I was using an iPad map as I hadn't yet got a Ghanaian sim for the phone and there were two towns with roughly the same name on the route. I chose the wrong one and by the time I discovered the error, it was dark. I turned into the nearest town, a beach resort called Busua and checked into a hotel. I was still feeling weak after the meltdown in Abidjan and rang Chloe, telling her I was lost. As always, she came up with a solution, phoning a contact who put me in touch with a chap called Sly who said he could drive me to Kumasi. I agreed as I was a little nervous about burning out the new clutch. However, Sly turned out to be a far worse driver than me, continuously stalling the van or accelerating in a series of jerks. It would have been better to have driven myself but despite that, we managed to reach Kumasi before Omotola, Rob and Jack.

I had some time to kill and as Kumasi was once the capital of the former Ashanti kingdom, one of Africa's mightiest empires, I was keen to do some sightseeing. As a military man, top of my list was the Kumasi Fort and Military Museum. Its exhibitions trace the evolution of the Gold Coast Regiment from the colonial era to the present-day Ghana Armed Forces. Of particular interest was the British Military Cemetery containing graves of those killed in the final Anglo–Ashanti clash. The Ashanti fought five wars against the British, winning or forcing a truce in most of them, but ultimately losing their empire after the War of the Golden Stool. The golden stool was the Ashanti royal throne; when Sir Frederick Mitchell Hodgson visited Kumasi in 1900, he queried why he, as Queen Victoria's envoy, was allocated an 'ordinary' seat and not the golden stool. He then ordered his men to find and seize the throne. This was a grave insult, provoking enraged warriors to attack Hodgson's men.

Vastly out-numbered, the British contingent, consisting of twenty-nine Britons and five hundred Nigerians, rapidly withdrew to a small stockade. They managed to hold off the Ashanti with six small field guns and four Maxim machine guns for several weeks until a rescue party of seven hundred men arrived. By this time, many of the starving fighters in the stockade were too ill to be evacuated and all the remaining food and ammunition stocks were left for them as the others

– including Hodgson, his wife and a hundred Nigerians – fled with their rescuers for the coast, chased by twelve thousand Ashanti warriors. Two Victoria Crosses were awarded in those epic battles, but as the Ashanti had not lost their sacred golden stool, they considered themselves victorious. Be that as it may, the Ashanti territories were incorporated into Ghana – known then as the Gold Coast colony – two years later.

I wish I could have delved deeper into Kumasi's fascinating past, but we had work to do and that evening I met up with Rob, Jack and Omotola. With her was a top Ghanaian neurologist, Dr Vida Obese, who would be in charge of our extremely busy itinerary and had arranged a host of press interviews. This involved getting up every morning at five to appear on breakfast TV, but it was worthwhile for the good it did.

Vida also runs clinics for Parkinson's patients and allowed us to sit in on her sessions. We met the husbands, wives and carers of those afflicted and in group discussions I told them why I was doing this journey and reassured them that they weren't alone. There were people throughout the world in our condition, I stressed, and one day there would be a cure, although probably not in our time.

It was interesting to see Vida in her element and what a good job she was doing. But no matter how hard she worked, it is still the tip of an iceberg. However, it is in no small measure thanks to her that there is far more awareness of the disease in Ghana than in most African countries.

A day or two later we left for the capital, Accra, where Omotola and I were scheduled to do more press interviews. I managed to take an evening off to visit Dan Frimpong, the brigadier general who had paved the way for a 'painless' visa application. Dan lived thirty minutes outside Accra but my driver got lost and it took longer than expected to get there. I had not brought enough Parkinson's pills and arrived in a bit of a heap.

Although now retired, Dan had commanded the Ghanaian Army's armoured vehicle unit and we had been on the same troop leaders' course at Bovington in 1985. It's not unusual for Commonwealth officers to be sent to Sandhurst or training centres such as Bovington and I got to know him quite well – although not as well as I would have liked. We reminisced at length and funnily enough one of his fondest memories was us having a few pints at a pub called the Brace of Pheasants in Plush, Dorchester. I found it strangely reassuring that here we were, forty years later, meeting up on Dan's home turf, talking about quaffing ales in a Dorset tavern. The close international contacts and networks formed by the British Army are simply incredible and it would be a sad day if those were lost.

Dan's wife had cooked supper, but without pills I was an inadequate guest and unable to eat, so they made up a doggy bag to take back to my hotel. Even in my depleted state, it was fantastic meeting up with an old friend again.

Between media sessions, I urgently needed to get a visa for Nigeria, which was proving to be a red tape headache. Rob and Jack were flying into Lagos and managed to get their visas relatively easily, but the embassy was not interested in granting a visa to travel through a land border.

I was becoming more and more frustrated, particularly as I was relying on Omotola, who was doing her best to expedite visas through her contacts in Nigeria and I somewhat foolishly remarked that she hadn't been doing a particularly good job. It was a flippant, off-the-cuff remark that was meant to be humorous as I knew she was doing her best, but she walked out in tears. I felt awful, running after her saying I was an insensitive old git and apologised profusely. She graciously accepted the abject apology but it was a low point in our relationship and I'm extremely grateful she forgave me and we managed to remain good friends.

It now seemed extremely unlikely that the Nigerian leg of the odyssey would happen, with Rob and Jack flying out in a couple of days and me without a visa. I don't like to ask for favours unless I have to, but in desperation contacted the British embassy to see if they could pull some strings. Ten minutes later my phone rang. It was the embassy. An official said if I went to the Nigerian consulate within the next half an hour, I would get a visa. It was 4.30 p.m. on a Friday and Jack and I sped off, clutching the necessary paperwork. The consulate was closed, but thanks to the British ambassador's intervention, a Nigerian official allowed us in through the back door.

There I got more bad news. I had filled in an airplane – not a vehicle – entry form. Consequently, I had to do it all again and come back the next morning with the correct paperwork. Finally, the visa was granted. Take it from me, the thump of that stamp on a passport is one of the most reassuring sounds in Africa.

Wasting no time, Rob and Jack caught a plane to Lagos while I drove to the border with Togo, heading directly for the capital, Lomé, on the coast. For some bizarre reason, I imagined it would be like Florida, with a promenade running along the oceanfront and lots of people on the beach. Instead, my satnav took me directly through the town centre, a large pedestrianised market area with umbrella-covered stalls spilling into the road. It was packed solid and at great inconvenience vendors had to move their stalls filled with sunglasses, flip-flops and other plastic bric-a-brac out of the way as I slowly squeezed through. There was no way I could reverse and had no option but to keep going. It was potentially a volatile situation so I locked the wagon's doors and wound up the windows, expecting a litany of angry outbursts. Fortunately, everyone seemed remarkably patient and good-natured about this obviously lost foreigner.

Eventually, I reached the beach and was looking for a bar that had been recommended on the iOverlander app, but instead found myself on a sand track surrounded by huts in a shanty village. It was like being back in the Sahara and, ever wary of getting stuck in the sand, I kept going until I saw a hotel where staff graciously allowed me to spend the night in the car park.

The next morning, I crossed the Mono River just before Togo's border with Benin and stopped at a guesthouse called

Hotel L'Oasis to have a cup of tea and take a photo of a cluster of brightly coloured fishing boats. While doing so, a stocky white man in colourful African print shirt and baggy shorts appeared. Just as surprisingly, he spoke perfect English with a slight South African drawl.

'Nick Hales,' he said, putting out his hand. 'I saw your van and the Parkinson's logo.'

It turned out he owned the hotel with his wife. We got chatting and he told me his sister-in-law had a neurological condition similar to Parkinson's. That's why he had been interested in the logo on the wagon. He then invited me for supper and to stay the night. All on the house – I was to be his guest.

'Sorry, I'm in a bit of a hurry,' I said, trying not to be discourteous. 'I have to get to Nigeria by midday tomorrow.'

'Don't worry. I'll get someone to take you to the border first thing in the morning. Please stay.'

It was an offer I couldn't refuse, and I'm glad I didn't. Nick's wife, Afia Mala, is a renowned Togolese singer, while Nick himself is one of those genuine adventurers one finds throughout Africa. He had been born on a Birmingham sink estate, but as a young boy moved to Zambia when his father found work in the copper mines. I later discovered he had written a book called *Life on the Edge*, vividly recounting hair-raising escapades from diving off oil rigs in the shark-infested Persian Gulf to receiving death threats from the Taliban and presiding over Voodoo ceremonies. He's certainly a colourful character.

As promised, Nick woke me early the next day and his driver escorted me to the border. From there, I drove through Benin as fast as I could, reaching Nigeria just before noon.

30

Nigeria

The Nigerian–Benin border was by far the busiest boundary I had crossed in Africa. In fact, with the shouting crowds and bustling traffic, it was chaos. No other word for it.

Suddenly, in the seething morass of people I spotted two Englishmen waving at me. My problems and confusion instantly disappeared as I shook hands with the 'two Tims' who had arrived a short while beforehand to ease my immigration procedures. I was only expecting one of them – Tim Hepworth – an ex-soldier doing security work in Nigeria who had offered to help me get into the country when I arrived. I would also be staying with him for the next month.

I cannot stress strongly enough the effort Tim expended on my behalf. He organised everything: transport to meetings, visits to various embassies, rounding up potential sponsors, gathering expats I might have met in the past and even inviting one of my squadron second-in-commands to dinner. Nothing was too much trouble and I laughed (something people with Parkinson's don't do much) more often than at any other point of the journey.

I had never met Tim, but by chance he had stumbled across me on the internet the day he learnt that a friend of his father's had Parkinson's. From then on, he made it his business to help me in any way he could. The unlimited and unconditional support that I received from people like Tim not only kept me going, but made me absolutely determined to reach Cape Town at the southern end of Africa.

The other Tim – Tim Illingworth – had been one of my platoon commanders at Harrogate a long time ago, although I had to confess to not remembering him well. I knew his parents much better, having first met his father Richard at Bovington in 1995. Richard suggested that it might be useful to touch base with his son in Nigeria. I probably made all the right noises but promptly forgot about it.

Luckily Richard had not, and warned his son that I was inbound and thank goodness he did. While Tim Hepworth made living in Lagos manageable and fun, Tim Illingworth made travelling safely in some very rough areas possible and I simply could not have gone further without his intervention and help. He worked for a private security company and had excellent contacts with the Nigerian police which would later pay dividends.

With Tim Hepworth leading the way, I was soon through customs and three hours later we were enjoying cold beers around the swimming pool in his gated community house.

Omotola, Rob and Jack had already flown in and, as this was Omotola's hometown, she would be in charge of our itinerary. Our hosts were the Adewunmi Desalu Parkinson's Foundation (ADPF), which supports Nigerians living with Parkinson's and provides drugs, shelter and accommodation. Adewunmi Desalu was a globally renowned Nigerian mathematician and engineer specialising in electronics and space technology, who valiantly fought the disease for ten years until his death in 2019. His wife Morin, a hugely respected Nigerian businesswoman in her own right, established the ADPF in his memory and it does fantastic work thanks to her extraordinary commitment and drive.

The foundation had just finished building a new centre in Lagos and our first press excursion was a one-and-a-half-mile walk by about 150 Parkinson's-afflicted people in the city centre. It was pouring with rain and our polyethylene capes did nothing to keep us dry, but the media was out in force and we held a very powerful press conference afterwards where some extremely brave people told their own harrowing stories of living with the disease.

Morin arranged TV and radio interviews ranging from serious chat shows with medical mandarins to trendy hip-hop DJ programmes, thus reaching an impressively diverse audience. Omotola was absolutely brilliant on air and I was very pleased that the talks focused on Parkinson's in general and not just my journey.

Nigeria is one of the most unequal countries in Africa, its society ranging from gated communities where people are so rich they don't know what to do with their money to shanties where people have no money at all. Rich and poor live cheek by jowl and it's possible to move from a highly affluent area into a slum merely by crossing a street. As a result, you have residential suburbs where houses cost north of half a million pounds a stone's throw from places like Makoko, the world's largest floating slum, where more than 200,000 people live in lean-to shacks and leaking boats on the Lagos Lagoon.

Like any city with extreme wealth disparity, Lagos can be exceptionally dangerous. Gangs of feral youths known as 'area boys' prowl the streets, robbing pedestrians and selling drugs. It's essential to have some local knowledge of which areas to avoid. Despite that, it's a vibrant city, heaving and muscling, trying to work out where it sits in the world. There's no doubt it's on course to be Africa's colossus and we were extraordinarily well looked after, wining and dining in nightclubs and restaurants that are world-class by any standards.

One club that really stood out for me was Sailor's, a live music restaurant built on stilts at the edge of the lagoon where Tim Hepworth, Rob and I went to soak up the music and enjoy the vibrancy of the city. On one occasion the androgynous MC was playing rap music – not my favourite choice – at such volume that I could barely hear myself speak and decided to leave early. As I shuffled out clutching the stair rail, somebody came up from behind and took my arm.

'Let me make sure you get down the stairs all right.'

I turned around and it was the MC, who had just finished her set. Her name was Kelsey and she turned out to be nothing like her hard, street-rapping, onstage persona. She was the most delightful person, genuinely concerned about this old git hobbling down the stairs trying not to topple over. When she heard my tale from Tim – he was always promoting me – she was quite overcome and gave me a huge hug. Her makeup was streaked with tears. She waited with us until our car arrived and made sure that I was safely inside. I had never met her before and probably never will again. But I'll never forget her.

It was soon time to move on, and my biggest concern now was trying to get diesel for the wagon. Nigeria has the tenth-largest oil reserves in the world, yet cars have to queue for fuel. Diesel is even more difficult to come by than petrol and Tim's driver had to scour garages around the city, filling up jerry cans wherever he found a few gallons. Nigeria's oil is concentrated in the 27,000-square-mile Niger Delta, an area headbutting into the Gulf of Guinea that makes the wild west seem tame. The delta has been teetering on anarchy for decades and it's estimated that a large percentage of the country's crude is stolen through criminal cartels variously made up of rogue soldiers, militant separatists and disgruntled oil company employees. Most of the theft is accomplished through the extremely dangerous acts of either 'hot tapping' – cutting into a pipeline and siphoning off oil – or 'cold tapping', where pipelines are simply blown up and the oil diverted. As a result of non-stop sabotage, oil spills have totally devastated fragile mangrove eco-systems and fish habitats and poisoned soil and groundwater, posing a serious threat to public health. In fact, the Niger Delta is the most polluted region in the world and an example of 'ecocide'.

Thanks to Tim's driver, we had enough diesel to reach Cameroon, but the next problem was my old nemesis, getting a visa. This time it was not obtuse embassies – in fact the Cameroon consular general, Manga Bessem Elizabeth, could not have been more helpful. However, she said she could not in good conscience grant me a visa as it was too dangerous. If I went through the north-east borders, I would likely encounter Boko Haram, Islamic militants who gained international notoriety by seizing schoolgirls as sex slaves. If I went south-east, I could be kidnapped by Cameroon's anglophone separatists. In Cameroon, it's known as '*Crise Anglophone*' (the 'anglophone crisis'), an ongoing civil war between the government and separatists from the country's English-speaking areas bordering Nigeria. On top of that, my van was worth a lot of money. So, if the fundamentalists and separatists didn't get me, bog-standard criminals probably would.

The situation looked grim and Tim Illingworth, who knew the situation better than most, agreed with the consular general, advising me to ship the wagon from Port Harcourt to Douala, Cameroon's largest port. But Port Harcourt was slap-bang in the crime-riddled Niger Delta and the campervan would have to be loaded onto a cargo ship by crane – out of my sight. There was no guarantee that a prized four-wheel-drive vehicle, fully loaded with expensive equipment, would arrive in Douala. I had no idea what to do and sat back, hoping some solution would miraculously emerge.

It did. While scanning iOverlander posts, I noticed that two travellers had safely got into Cameroon through the border between the towns of Gembu (Nigeria) and Banyo (Cameroon). This is a minor crossing conveniently sited between the areas of activity of Boko Haram and the anglophone separatists, as neither group shows much interest in this almost impassable route. I managed to persuade the consular general that I could also get through there, and she reluctantly stamped my passport. As an added precaution, she arranged for a Cameroonian army escort to meet me in Banyo.

By now the monsoon rains had arrived with a vengeance and Tim decided to accompany me to the country's capital, Abuja,

450 miles away. He brought an escort vehicle and a driver with him and also hired a unit of the Nigerian Mobile Police.

I'd had new front shocks fitted in Lagos and the wagon was running beautifully. The road snaked through spectacular hilly countryside and, despite the dire predictions, I didn't feel unsafe at all. It took two days to reach Abuja and, after spending the night in the capital, Tim returned to Lagos.

The driver and I continued with the police to Gembu along an excellent dual carriageway which diminished to a track as we neared the border. Finding the best road to Gembu was tricky as landslides had closed the obvious route, but we made our way to a hotel where we would spend our last night in Nigeria. There we got directions to the emigration and police posts and were told in no uncertain terms that we were in for a hell of a ride. I also noticed that all vehicles in the area were serious, heavy-duty, off-roaders and there were more than a few abandoned as scrap on the side of the road. Equally ominous was the fact that there was only one other entry in the emigration log before me – not to mention a somewhat bemused crowd gathering to see us off.

Once our passports had been stamped out of Nigeria, the tracks already churned up into a viscous slush by the pouring rain got steadily worse. In fact, in some places it wasn't even a track, just patches of flattened, soaked grass without markers and I had no idea if we were heading in the right direction. Only experienced transport drivers braved this quagmire using their mighty Pinzgauers – high-mobility, all-terrain utility vehicles – or rugged Series 3 Land Rovers that were so old the paint had peeled off. Most of the tyres on these classic workhorses were completely smooth and I wondered how they managed to grip in the glutinous mud. There is no doubt that these drivers were superb off-roaders – among the best I'd ever come across.

Sadly, my driver wasn't one of them. He was far more suited to negotiating the traffic jams of Lagos than extreme wildernesses. The worse the tracks got, the more he tried to compensate by flooring the accelerator. I remonstrated with him, but he refused to listen, gunning the engine for all its worth. Unfortunately, one of the more debilitating effects of Parkinson's is that it makes you take the path of least resistance rather than asserting yourself. If I had ordered him to stop, deflated the tyres to 20 p.s.i. and offloaded the heavy equipment weighing down the wagon into the empty police escort truck, we would have got through. These were things I knew well from years of off-road driving in conditions just as bad as this. It was second nature. All that was needed was a cool head, which sadly I did not have.

Instead, I sat back and hoped for the best – the worst possible option – and I still get angry when I think of what happened next. There was a Land Rover stuck in front of us, blocking the slippery track. Once again, ignoring all instructions, the driver accelerated madly and somehow skidded past the stranded vehicle, spraying mud and sliding precariously off the edges of the track.

We had got through, but more by fluke than anything else. Immediately afterwards we reached a river, about fifty yards wide and thigh-deep, judging by the villagers who were in the water waiting to help push. We managed to barge our way across, but my relief was short-lived. The track up the other bank was very wet and the wagon slipped into a gully. Once again, the driver tried to solve the problem by gunning the engine, but all that achieved was futile wheel-spinning.

Then suddenly the engine started over-revving wildly, a sound I now knew all too well. The driver had burnt out the clutch. And it was only two months since the Abidjan nightmare.

We were now well and truly stuck in no man's land. The only option was to get a tow truck – or rather a truck that could tow – to pull me to the Cameroon border about forty miles away. But where would I find one in the middle of one of the roughest wildernesses? Unlike the Ivory Coast, there was no Papi to come to my aid.

However, there was a village ahead where some of the transport drivers lived. Hoping against hope to find someone there to help, I locked up the wagon, paid someone to guard it, and set off in the police escort truck.

It seemed my luck was in, as a villager pointed to the house of someone who claimed to run a recovery operation. 'Claimed' was the operative word, as basically all he had was a six-wheeler Pinzgauer with some wire rope. We agreed on a fee, but had further problems as some of my dollars were considered out of date by the Central Bank of Nigeria. Fortunately, I had enough valid cash to cover the costs. The operation began but I feared the worst as he tied a simple bowline to connect two hefty vehicles.

It was harrowing in the extreme. The driver refused to listen when I told him to keep the rope taut and the wagon was viciously jerked each time he took up the slack. Luckily, I had fitted a steel bar to the front of the vehicle, which meant the shock impacted mainly on the solid chassis, but eventually even that was bent.

Gradually, minute by torturous minute, inch by miniscule inch, the Pinzgauer dragged the wagon up a never-ending array of slippery hills. Once at the top, the six-wheeler slewed down almost liquefied mud slopes with the wagon corkscrewing behind. Two days later, after a night spent outside a military checkpoint, I saw the border post ahead. It had taken us three days to get there, an average of thirteen miles a day.

As arranged by the Cameroonian embassy, gendarmes were waiting for me, which was surprising as I was forty-eight hours late.

It had been an adventure all right, and one I would rather not repeat. But at least I was now in Cameroon – and for the first time since leaving Liberia, turned south towards the tip of the continent.

But even better, I had made it without bumping into Boko Haram or *Crise Anglophone* fighters.

31

Cameroon

Getting across the border did not mean I was out of the woods – either metaphorically or physically. I still had a crippled car that wasn't going anywhere under its own steam.

There was not much I could do except negotiate another fee with the Pinzgauer driver to tow the wagon to Banyo, now about forty miles away. My misfortune was proving lucrative for him, but no one could deny that he was there when I needed him.

The road to Banyo was slightly better, as it was rocky rather than muddy, but even so, the abused tow rope eventually snapped during one particularly nasty jolt. We re-tied the two vehicles but the rope was now only six feet long and it required intense concentration not to slam into the back of the Pinzgauer.

Banyo was a reasonably sized town. The tow driver dropped me and the wagon off outside the police station, where I was greeted by a gendarme *capitaine* dressed immaculately in his finest no. 2 uniform. No doubt he was expecting a British Army colonel and I can only imagine his surprise when he saw this scruffy specimen emerging from a battered and bent, mud-splattered vehicle. Nonetheless, he was charming and showed me to the hotel where I would be staying while waiting for a tow to Foumbot, the next town, where someone from the

British embassy was waiting. Now resigned to my fate, I started enjoying this part of the adventure as the hotel was comfortable, I was fed and watered and it was pleasant wandering around the town watching kids playing football and people going about their daily business.

The main problem was that there were no proper tow trucks in Banyo. The police helped as much as they could and we tracked down a man with a cattle lorry. It was far from ideal, with high wooden sides to keep the cows in and a rotten plank floor, but it was the only show in town. It didn't have ramps, so to load the wagon onto the back required some creative thinking.

Fortunately, there was a retaining wall near the road. We towed the wagon on to it, reversed the lorry below and then – using two planks as ramps and with some energetic shoving – I steered the wagon onto the truck bed. To say it was a tight fit was understating the case; I barely made it without mangling my wing mirrors. Once loaded, I couldn't open the front doors due to the cattle rails and had to climb over the driver's seat and squeeze out through the side sliding door.

I thought the driver would strap the wagon down, but instead he merely deflated all four tyres, which I thought was a dumb idea. It would hardly stop the wagon from being slammed around every time we hit a pothole.

We set off at about 8 p.m. – me, the driver and his teenage assistant. Foumbot was about fifty miles south, but as the road was slippery and potholed, we rarely exceeded fifteen miles an hour. It was slow but hardly leisurely as the constant cranking and banging – either the lorry's ancient suspension groaning or the wagon bouncing around – frayed my nerves. I tried to console myself by thinking that as long as the van's windscreen didn't shatter, which would be almost impossible to replace locally, I would be OK. If the wing mirrors broke, I could fix them with strips of metal and any dents would be more of a cosmetic than a functional problem. Suffice it to say that my heart was continuously in my mouth as we clunked over rocks, forest debris and ruts and endured the inconvenience of regular stops at police checkpoints in the militant anglophone separatist area.

After almost three days, we chugged into Foumbot where, to my dismay, I found that the British embassy representative had got tired of waiting and had left. Once again, I was stranded. Big problem for me, but not so much for the cattle truck driver. For another exorbitant fee, he would take me to the capital city of Cameroon, Yaoundé.

'OK, but you have to find a cashpoint,' I said.

No problem. He drove the big vehicle down some narrow streets in the middle of town, stopped outside an ATM and I withdrew wads of money. I also checked the wagon to find that amazingly the flat tyres trick had worked perfectly. The wagon was not only undamaged – it didn't have a single dent. Well, not a new one anyway.

Just as I breathed a huge sigh of relief I noticed that one of the wagon's wheels was sticking out of the bottom of the flatbed. The weight of the van had been too much for a section of rotten planking and broken through. We needed to fix this urgently in case the entire bed collapsed.

We pulled into a trucker's stop to replace the broken plank. I knew how to do this with wooden blocks and strategically placed jacks, but didn't have the authority to order the driver and his helper around. They were eager, but hopelessly inefficient and couldn't get the levers and angles right. Whenever I tried to intervene, they wouldn't listen. As a result, it took us all night to get everything in the right position, jack the wagon up and replace the broken section with planks from another lorry. Despite that, I was enjoying my time with these tough Cameroonians in the outback. They lived a hard life, but always seemed cheerful.

We set off for the capital, about 190 miles away, and the road started improving dramatically. Our average speed was now into double figures and we were going along merrily when we were stopped at another of the ubiquitous police roadblocks.

However, as bad luck would have it, a particularly officious policeman was in charge. He said, with the trademark self-importance of a petty official, that my driver's lorry was only registered to carry food and livestock, not another vehicle. This was the first time the driver had heard of such a law, if one existed but, despite our remonstrations, the policeman refused to let us travel further.

I rang the British embassy and got through to a Royal Marine captain. He spoke directly to the policeman, saying I was expected at the embassy and any prevention of this could result in a diplomatic incident. I also tried to act the part, pretending that I was far more important than I actually was. The policeman shook his head. We could go no further.

While this was happening a car coming at speed from the other side of the road failed to see the checkpoint and smashed into the barriers, careering into the bush. There was much yelling and excitement and in the confusion I said to my driver, 'Let's get out of here!'

He agreed, and the three of us jumped into the lorry and eased off as unobtrusively as possible.

We arrived at Yaoundé at midnight and were met by a group of Gurkha security staff who guided us to an apartment block where a British military detachment was based. Cameroon is part of the Commonwealth with close ties to the UK armed forces and, thanks to the extremely helpful embassy, I would be staying with the British liaison contingent over the next few weeks. The next day a conventional recovery truck offloaded the wagon from the cattle lorry and took it to a garage that maintained the fleet of embassy vehicles. My genial driver and his teenage sidekick then left for the long drive back to Banyo, hopefully this time avoiding officious policemen.

I knew I would not be able to source a clutch in Cameroon and had already contacted Rob Willis at Volkstrek to get a new one. But to get it from Aberystwyth in Wales to Cameroon was the next hurdle.

Fortunately, an embassy employee was flying to Yaoundé from Heathrow and if Rob could get the clutch to her in London, she would bring it out. Rob's a brilliant bloke and did exactly that. The embassy staffer stuffed the parts into her hand luggage, just as Hank had done when I was in Abidjan and, by the end of the following week, the wagon was good to go.

My time was not wasted while waiting. I did a lot of Parkinson's awareness work – probably more so than in any other city. The embassy was superb, organising press interviews and arranging a meeting with Cameroon's chief medical officer and a visit to the neurological hospital, where I spoke to patients and neurologists and even someone recovering from brain surgery. Impressive stuff anywhere, let alone in a country where resources are limited.

Also, through Parkinson's Africa, I met Hilaire Roger, an indomitable inspiration who had founded the Parkinson's Cameroon Support group. He has severely advanced Parkinson's, but still does incredible work campaigning for those afflicted. His commitment to the cause is total and he will speak to anyone who will listen and bang on any door if necessary. At times it was poignantly painful to hear him give speeches as he stammered terribly but continued undaunted until the words came out. His unconquerable optimism and positiveness, despite the terrible curved ball thrown at him, was beyond remarkable. Through him I met many Cameroonians living with Parkinson's and at one conference I addressed about 150 people. He introduced me by saying how lucky they were that I had come all this way specifically to visit them. While not strictly true, that certainly gilded my journey.

However, my time was rapidly running out. I had a deadline to meet Rob in Libreville to shoot more film and I'd already been far longer in Cameroon than anticipated.

Once the wagon was ready, I headed south for Gabon. It was a pleasant drive and I was ultra-cautious with the clutch. I don't think many drivers can claim to have burnt out two in as many months. There was a lone customs official at the border who let me through cheerfully and once in the country I marvelled at the stunning scenery. Tree foliage formed a spectacular arch over the road and the luxuriant bush glistened with every shade of vibrant green imaginable.

Soon after the border I passed through a village and noticed people waving and shouting at me. Thinking I had unwittingly driven through a police checkpoint or done something wrong, I quickly stopped and got out.

It was the complete opposite. The villagers were actually urging me to stop for refreshments. The chief himself invited me to join him and that evening I sat around the fire with his friends, drinking beer and spinning yarns. I told them about my journey and Parkinson's and they were very receptive. The chief then allowed me to park the wagon outside his house and spend the night there. This is what I'd always imagined travelling in Africa would be like.

The next morning, I set off for Libreville and, just as I was marvelling at how smooth the road was, I hit a pothole. In fact, two, as I bounced out of the first pothole straight into another, even bigger one, skidding wildly off into the bush before regaining control and veering back onto the road. The wagon then ground to a halt.

I got out to find the wheel hub twisted at a forty-five-degree angle. This was serious and I suspected that my shock absorbers, which had been replaced in Lagos and weren't the best, had collapsed. I was wondering what to do when a well-dressed chap in a Toyota Hilux stopped and asked if I needed help. I certainly did. As we were surveying the problem, a massive articulated logging truck stopped and the driver also came to assist.

It was now dark and the chap in the Hilux went to fetch a mechanic from the village I had just passed through. While waiting, the truck driver – who told me his name was Gloria

(I had to ask him to repeat that) – built a fire to ward off the forest animals. Sceptical at first, I was glad he did as the bush seethed with wildlife. I could hear elephants trumpeting and there were a lot of monkeys. We chewed the fat about how beautiful Gabon was and he said it was a pity about the potholes. I told him this was one of the better roads I had driven on.

A couple of hours later the Hilux driver and the mechanic arrived. The five of us (the lorry driver's assistant had joined us to help) took the wheel off and fiddled around with the suspension, trying to fix the bent shock absorber. It took seven hours to semi-straighten it with some hefty levering until at last I could drive off to get proper help. The chaps remained with me the whole time and it was after midnight when we left in convoy to the next village, me following the logging truck and the Hilux behind, going slowly as even a minor bump could again cripple the wagon. This demanded extra-careful driving, but I was so exhausted, particularly as I'd forgotten to take my pills, that I slipped into a bit of a funk, unable to concentrate. I signalled to Gloria to stop, saying I couldn't carry on. Somewhat exasperated, he got into the wagon and drove the rest of the way, while his sixteen-year-old sidekick drove the articulated vehicle. This was extremely impressive – most kids his age can't even handle an automatic street car and here this youngster was, confidently getting behind the wheel of a multi-wheeled, 33-tonne logging truck.

Two hours later we arrived at a village called Lalara, little more than a logging camp at a junction where the main road splits to Libreville and Mitzic, and I parked outside the local mechanic's workshop. The next morning both Gloria and the Hilux driver popped around before leaving to see if I was all right. I could not thank them enough.

The bush mechanic's workshop was a mud-floored tin hut with rudimentary shelves crammed with tools and used spare parts. A socket connected to the streetlight outside was the sole source of electricity. This was grass roots engineering at its finest. He whipped the wheels off and said he could easily fix the problem – but despite the thousands of spare parts cluttering his shop's shelves, he unfortunately did not have the Volkswagen brand. I would have to source those parts myself.

But where? I only had one contact, a well-known fixer in Libreville called Marcel, who had been highly recommended, but was unfortunately not always highly reliable. Especially at locating motor spares.

However, it was imperative that I make it to Libreville as Rob had just arrived and I needed to make the most of his time. With our limited budget, we had to get to work filming right away and I was persuaded against my will to catch a taxi to Libreville as soon as possible. As a firm believer in the old army adage never to get separated from your kit, I was extremely reluctant to leave the wagon behind with a total stranger. It was totally against my better judgment.

The taxi arrived at about ten the following night. I grabbed a bag, handed the wagon's keys to the mechanic and left for the capital. The driver was chewing *khat* – a stimulant with effects similar to, but less powerful than, amphetamine or speed – and there was no doubt he was high. He zoomed off down the road at breakneck speed and when not babbling on his phone, to my absolute astonishment he was watching film clips on it! There was one other passenger, Ali, who seemed to know the driver, while I silently sat back and hoped for the best.

About an hour outside Libreville, police stopped us at a roadblock. The driver handed over his papers and I could tell straight away by the frown creasing the policeman's face that there were problems. 'Your car details are incorrect,' he said.

The driver protested vehemently, but to no avail. The vehicle was impounded.

'What about us?' I asked.

The police thought about that for a moment and agreed they could not just leave us on the side of the road at midnight. They took Ali and me to the police station and allocated some floor space in the jail. Fortunately, the door was not locked.

The next day we were told we would have to find our own way to Libreville, but at least we got a ride to the main road. We tried hitching. Ali was carrying a huge bag of rags – for what, I have no idea – and there was no chance of any motorist giving us a lift. Eventually, we caught a bus.

Two hours later Ali, who by now was a friend, made sure that I was safely dropped off at the Tropicana Hotel where I was scheduled to meet Rob and Marcel.

I was strangely despondent. All I could think of was my wagon left unlocked in a strange village.

32

Gabon – Spirits of the Forest

Gabon is among the most beautiful countries in Africa, with lush rainforests, glorious beaches, lagoons and estuaries. I should have been having the time of my life.

But as I have said before, travelling in Africa is like playing snakes and ladders, with the ladders far shorter than the snakes. You don't play to win; you play to enjoy an exciting game. For anyone travelling overland, that's the best bit of advice I can give.

In Gabon, the ladders turned out to be even shorter than usual, more through circumstances than anything else. For a start, our fixer Marcel was unfortunately a little short of solutions in this particular game. He certainly had connections in high places, but as he was in much demand, we seemed to be low on his list of priorities – especially with regards to the wagon. All my worldly possessions were in the van and I needed to get it to Libreville right away. Marcel kept promising it would arrive shortly on a flatbed truck but despite my urging, nothing happened. Every day, I simply got a shrug and the answer, 'Soon'. It was totally out of my control and I had dire visions of the trusty wagon being sold off and never seeing it again.

The main focus of the Gabon section of the odyssey was to explore specific medicines known only to the Pygmy forest tribes. These incredible people believe that the jungle has remedies for almost every ailment imaginable – even for Parkinson's. Yet whenever we tried to get Marcel to arrange meetings with healers, he either cancelled or rescheduled. And this was the reason I had rushed down from Lalara, leaving the wagon in the care of someone I hardly knew and could barely contact due to a sporadic mobile signal.

Despite Marcel's disorganisation, we did manage to get some filming done. I had been given the name of a French anthropologist, Hugues Obiang Poitevin, who'd done extensive studies on Gabonese forest medicines. Rob filmed him as he told me that the core ingredient is the drug ibogaine obtained from the iboga shrub, which has huge spiritual significance to the forest dwellers. Native to the West and Central African rainforests, iboga's yellowish root bark is an exceptionally strong hallucinogenic and, according to the Pygmy healers, an iboga cleansing process physically dumps all the rubbish in your brain, curing diseases and mentally taking your mind to places where you can start again.

However, to see this first-hand, the Frenchman, who looked more like a hippie than an anthropologist, said we needed to witness a *Bwiti* ceremony. That lies at the heart of the relationship between Gabonese Pygmies and the forest, where iboga is taken for both religious and health reasons. This should have been relatively simple to organise, but once again, Marcel kept changing plans at the last moment.

Nothing seemed to be going right and all the while our expenses were skyrocketing. Rob had flown from London at significant cost and we were staying in an upmarket hotel, so each day we didn't spend filming was a day wasted. A further aggravating factor was the trouble we were having arranging a visa for my son Wilfred, who was going to help drive through Congo-Brazzaville and the DRC. Wilfred was crucial to the next stage of the journey – two of the potentially more hazardous areas – and it was imperative he got that entry permit.

At the same time, I was getting lots of long-distance, not terribly helpful, advice on where my daughter Millie should join us in Africa. She was coming soon and these knotty, interrelated problems were stressing me out, severely intensifying my Parkinson's trigger points. The weather was bloody hot as well. I found myself incapable of getting out of my bed on more occasions than I care to remember. The challenges ahead of me looked almost insurmountable.

At this low point we met Jannie Fourie, manager of an eco-tourist resort company, who told us that one of their lodges was empty and invited us to stay. A South African, he was a tremendous bloke, but I don't think he realised what a lifesaver his offer was. His resort, Pongara, was across the bay from Libreville and famous for viewing elephants emerging from the forest and frolicking in the surf – just the break I needed.

Unfortunately, we didn't see swimming elephants, but halfway through our stay I got tremendous news. My van was at last on its way back to Libreville and the recovery vehicle would deliver it to the hotel. I needed to be there to make sure it wasn't left in the street.

By a stroke of extraordinarily good luck, Jannie knew an excellent mechanic called Moses, who came back with us to the hotel armed with little more than a bag of spanners and a handkerchief. My relief on seeing the van was palpable and it seemed that all my possessions were still intact.

While Moses was tinkering around, I filmed him on FaceTime and Rob Willis, who was watching on his phone several thousand miles away in Aberystwyth, suddenly remarked, 'Guy, that looks like a crack in the engine mount block.'

I looked closely, then saw it; a great big fracture in the block mounting the engine onto the chassis. My heart sank. It looked serious.

'No, we can fix it,' Rob said. 'I just have to find the correct block.'

It took him almost two days, but once again the ever-reliable Rob magnificently came up trumps, sourcing the last available engine mount in the UK from a supplier in Bournemouth. However, it was Friday and the garage was about to close for the weekend, so Elle – Wilfred's girlfriend – drove all the way to the Dorset coast to fetch it from a hiding place outside the shop, while Wilfred drove to Wales to get other parts we needed from Rob. The way the three of them managed to coordinate that in such a short time was miraculous.

Wilfred flew out to Gabon the next day, but while he was on the plane, I got some startling news. His visa had been rejected. And I had paid Marcel a lot of money to get that precious visa. I very rarely lose my temper, but I was now livid. I immediately phoned Marcel. There was no answer at first. Eventually, after about an hour, he picked up.

'What's this about Wilfred's visa being rejected?' I demanded.

'Don't you worry. I'll get him another one at the airport,' he said sheepishly.

'No – listen to me. I am *very* worried – and *you* had better worry. I can't fix my van if he doesn't get through. Go to the airport now and sort this mess out.'

I don't think Marcel had ever heard anyone that angry and when I arrived at the airport he was already there. He had an airside airport pass so could go into restricted areas, where he met Wilfred and duly got him an entry visa at the immigration desk. It cost even more money.

The relief at seeing Wilfred and getting the spare parts was overwhelming and my Parkinson's funk dissipated. At last the journey was back on track, but as my three-week Gabonese visa was starting to run out, I had to move fast.

After delivering the spare parts to Moses, we got more good news. Marcel had finally managed to organise a *Bwiti* for us in a village near the capital. We were the only visitors and Rob did a lot of filming with me speaking and dancing with the forest people.

It was fascinating in the extreme, the ceremony peaking when the forest *Ngangas* – spiritual healers – offered to give me some iboga that I could take on film. I was initially tempted, but the more I considered it, the more I thought it would be a bad idea. Iboga causes users to collapse and it's vital to have experienced healers around to assist while in this extreme hallucinogenic state. For me it was a step too far.

Despite that, I firmly believe there is something profoundly beneficial in the medicines found naturally in rainforests. As both quinine, a cure for malaria, and the origins of aspirin derive from plants, there is no reason why cures for critical diseases such as cancer, not to mention Parkinson's, shouldn't also be available in nature. I don't pretend to have stumbled across a Parkinson's cure, but I am convinced we should also be exploring natural remedies rather than relying solely upon chemical solutions supplied by the big pharmaceutical corporations.

With the *Bwiti* ceremony on film, it was now time to move on. However, to paraphrase the biblical proverb, 'Man plans and God laughs,' we then discovered that Wilfred had just three days left on his Gabon visa. We had applied for a fourteen-day visa, but for some reason, it was only valid for a week. Once again, more snakes than ladders.

As it was impossible to get Wilfred's visa extended in time, we decided to make the most of his remaining days and he would drive with me to Ndendé, the last proper village in Gabon before the Congo-Brazzaville border.

It was a brilliant trip, and one of the highlights of my life was crossing the equator twenty-seven miles south of Libreville with my son. Wilfred has a genuine spirit of adventure and is a great travelling companion. He's also extremely useful mechanically, as I found out when we heard a strange clunking noise coming from the wheel station. Wilfred removed the wheel, crawled under the van, and found that, despite Moses's excellent job, a bolt was missing from a brake calliper. As this could prove problematic later, we called the local mechanic who arrived with a sack of random nuts and bolts and, after much rummaging around, found one that fitted well enough.

Wilfred caught a bus back to Libreville the next day and I could barely control my emotions while saying goodbye. Not only would I miss my son as a fine companion, I needed him to help me drive as I feared the next section would be the worst of the odyssey. I would now have to do it on my own and, watching the clouds of dust billowing as the bus left, I have seldom felt so despondent. In fact, if I could have quit the odyssey honourably at that stage, I would have done so. It was the only time I felt like that, and thank goodness, it passed.

I got into the van, turned right and headed south.

Fortunately, I was now ahead of the rains. It would not have been possible to have driven on those roads in the monsoons, and I had to crack on to keep ahead.

My funk started to lift as I approached Congo-Brazzaville. The warm weather was perfect, the road challenging but not impossible, the scenery panoramic and I didn't see another car for close on six hours. My only sadness was Wilfred was not with me. He would have loved it.

To my relief, crossing into Congo-Brazzaville went smoothly, and I carried on towards Dolisie, the country's third-largest city. On the outskirts I stopped at a Total petrol station, filled up the wagon and asked the cashier if I could stop in the car park and have a sleep as I'd been driving all night. She nodded and also let me use the staff shower. An incredibly kind person, she recognised something was not quite right, so I told her I had Parkinson's and would be fine later. She asked where I was going and I said either Brazzaville or Pointe-Noire, as I could get an Angolan visa in either city. She said that if I went to Pointe-Noire, the hub of the country's oil industry and only a hundred miles away, her brother Jofran would drive me.

After I'd had a quick rest, Jofran arrived and chauffeured me to a restaurant on the Pointe-Noire beachfront called Brasserie de la Mer. It had been recommended by iOverlander as it had a car park where I could sleep and chill out while deciding what to do next.

To get to Angola, I had two options: I could either head directly south through Cabinda – an oil-rich enclave belonging to Angola but cut off by the DRC – or I could head east into the interior, crossing into a much wider area of the DRC. Cabinda was the significantly shorter route as it eliminated most of the DRC section, but it had a violent reputation. In 2010, separatist guerrillas shot up a bus carrying the Togo football team on its way to Luanda for the Africa Cup of Nations, killing three people and injuring several others.

However, when I heard that the inland road was worse than the Gembu–Banyo stretch where I – or at least my Nigerian driver – had burnt out the clutch, I opted to take my chances through Cabinda. The problem was that no one at the Angolan embassy seemed to know whether a single-entry visa into Cabinda would be valid for Angola as well. If not, I would have to get a second visa in Kinshasa, arguably Africa's most chaotic city and something I wanted to avoid at all costs.

I arrived at the Cabinda crossing to find that even the border officials didn't know the answer to the visa question. However, a fixer there told me that if I contributed a hundred dollars to the 'policeman's ball' – a quaint euphemism for a bribe – a single visa would indeed be valid for both entry points. The immigration official, knowing about my 'contribution', stamped my Cabinda entry a couple of pages away from the visa stamp on my passport to make the visa look 'unused' when I arrived at the Angola proper crossing. I thought that would solve the problem, but just as I was leaving, another official warned me to get a new visa for Angola. Who knew who was right?

Cabinda was an excellent choice, as the road was straight and, six hours later, I arrived at the DRC border without having been shot at by separatists.

There was nothing but endless scrub and sandy tracks in that particular stretch of the DRC, so I headed straight for Boma. The town had a dodgy reputation and I hurriedly bought some street food and followed the road towards the 1,710-foot Matadi Bridge spanning the mighty Congo River. It's a spectacular sight, until recently the longest suspension bridge in Africa and one of my bucket list destinations. It didn't disappoint when I arrived at 3 a.m., pausing to watch dawn breaking magnificently over the world's third-largest river by discharge volume.

Soon afterwards I saw a sign saying 'Angola' and expected the border to be about five miles away. But as I reached the top of the next hill, there it was, right in front of me. I planned to rest for a while, but the DRC customs officials hurried me through and before I knew it, the dreaded run through the two Congos was over. And far from being the worst section, it had been great fun.

33

Angola and Zambia

At the Angolan border, I was somewhat anxious about whether my Cabinda-issued visa – and donation to the… ahem, 'policeman's ball' – would work. My misgivings grew while being kept waiting for an hour. Then I heard the comforting 'thud' of a rubber stamp on a passport page. I was through.

The visa was valid for ten days, but as I had already used three of those getting through Cabinda and the DRC, I only had a week left. Somewhere along the line I would have to get a new visa, which actually fitted nicely with my plans as my daughter Millie and her friend Thomasina Bowyer-Bower were coming out. Initially, I wanted them to join me in Angola but, as misinformed friends and family in England believed that would be too dangerous, I changed the plan. I would instead fly to Zambia and meet them there. Zambia might seem to be far out of the way east, but I was also keen to interview Guy Scott, a former Zambian president who had Parkinson's and lived in Lusaka. This necessitated having a break in Zambia which, in retrospect, I badly needed. I would be able to renew my Angolan visa at the same time – they can usually only be obtained from outside the target country.

I had a more immediate problem to deal with, a strange crunching noise from the wagon's prop shaft that was getting louder. It worried me intensely as I knew the roads in northern Angola were terrible. The vehicle was still going so I could carry on and see what happened, but the risks of long-term damage and perhaps a ruined gearbox were too great. I decided to play it safe and find a recovery truck to take the wagon to the capital city Luanda where it could be fixed properly.

Just as in Banyo, the small Angolan border town of Noqui did not exactly have a fleet of AA-type recovery vehicles available. I drove down the hill into the ramshackle town centre and saw a man with his car bonnet up and tinkering with the engine. I asked him in my best French and English if there was a mechanic or recovery vehicle in the area, but he clearly didn't understand a word. He only spoke Portuguese. Two street youths sort of understood the gist of my question and gave me a lift on a motorbike back to the border. There they pointed to a couple of flatbed logging trucks.

With much gesticulating and me speaking in loud English, the logging drivers – who also only spoke Portuguese – indicated they could indeed take the wagon to Luanda. It was going to be expensive, but I decided that would still be cheaper than risking major mechanical repairs.

As in Banyo, there were no ramps to load the wagon, so the driver guided me down the road to a mound of earth, signalling I should drive up and he would reverse the flatbed beneath. He backed up as far as he could, but there was still a six-foot gap between the wagon and the truck. The two drivers borrowed bits of wood and made a makeshift ramp, which slipped at a crucial stage, leaving the wagon with a wheel suspended half off the flatbed. It was potentially a disaster waiting to happen, but I slowly managed to inch the van backwards while the drivers inserted more planks.

We were ready to go.

What I wasn't prepared for was how vast Angola is. It's huge and for the next three days we bumped along rutted dirt tracks, sometimes paradoxically going inland while Luanda is on the coast. Fortunately, there was a bed in the back of the cab so, despite the loud Angolan music, I slept when not keeping the amiable drivers company upfront.

I phoned the British ambassador, Roger Stringer, to brief him of my Parkinson's mission and he told me to come to the embassy. As usual, I would be arriving late at night, and he said he would be waiting but stressed we must use the bottom gate on the coastal road as the embassy is at the top of the highest hill in central Luanda. I explained that to the driver, but it got lost in translation and the next thing I knew he was following his satnav directions up a steeply winding, narrow lane in the sixteen-wheel, articulated truck. Somehow we made it. When Roger came out to meet us at about midnight, I'm sure the last thing he expected was to see a high VW van on a logging truck at the top of the city's main beacon. Anyway, he was pretty relaxed about it.

Next problem was how to offload the wagon. We needed a type of platform to reverse-engineer our loading method. Neither I nor the driver knew of any, but one of the embassy staff told us about an old factory warehouse which might be suitable. He was right. The warehouse had a loading platform, but only for static goods. There was no road to drive the wagon away once unloaded.

However, it was our only option. The driver reversed the truck up to the platform and I manoeuvred the wagon off, then had to execute a sixteen-point turn before bumping down a flight of concrete stairs onto the ground. I fervently thanked Rob Willis for fitting the armour plate protecting the underbelly of the wagon, which absorbed the bumps without even getting dented.

From there I drove the van to Sammy, a wonderful Lebanese mechanic who spoke good English and he soon pinpointed the problem. The prop shaft bearings and spline joint were worn as the holding bracket had been repeatedly broken. Sammy couldn't get the required parts, but thought he could make 'a plan' if necessary. It was time – yet again – to ring Volkstrek and speak to Rob Willis, who said he would try and get me one and have it flown out – as we had with the two clutches and other spares. Until then, the wagon would stay at Sammy's garage and I headed back to the embassy to book my ticket to Zambia.

The UK embassy in Luanda is a wonderful building, about 130 years old and built on the site of the original British representative's house in what was then a Portuguese colony. The representative's main job was to report the comings and goings of foreign ships – hence its location at the top of the hill alongside the four-hundred-year-old St Michael's fort. The ambassador's residence and other accommodation were inside the fortified compound, including a transit flat where I was allowed to stay. Roger, coincidentally an ex-Army officer (we had friends in common), was impressed by what I was doing and wanted to help in any way. His hospitality was magnificent; one night he asked what I would like for supper, and I heard myself saying – genuinely but with no expectations – that I would love a fish finger sandwich. To my astonishment, he replied that his kids also liked fish fingers and he had some in his fridge. The sandwich was superb and, although a small gesture, it was typical of how staff at all British embassies (apart from the Ivory Coast) went out of their way to help.

In the embassy garden is an impressive tree under which the missionary-explorer David Livingstone spent two months recovering from a near-fatal bout of malaria in 1854. As it happened, I was sitting under that same tree 168 years later when I also caught the mosquito-borne disease – although I didn't know it at the time. I obviously was aware something was wrong, alternating between fits of shaking fever and then feeling fine, but thought it was just another Parkinson's-related ailment. I should have known that fever spikes are a classic malaria symptom as I'd had it while in the regiment.

However, my Angolan visa was about to expire and I was scheduled to meet Millie and Thomasina in a few days' time, so had to leave for Zambia right away. The flight went through Johannesburg where I had to sprint clumsily around the large Oliver Tambo airport to catch the connecting shuttle to Lusaka. I got on board just in time, hot and sweaty, and feeling extremely ill.

When the plane landed I could barely stand but luckily a good Samaritan helped me off, getting me through immigration and carrying my luggage. I have no idea who he was, just a random stranger helping someone through the innate goodness of their heart.

Meeting me at the airport was Angus Mackie, who no doubt got a shock when he saw me stumbling and jabbering incoherently and he poured me into his car. As soon as we arrived at the house, Angus's wife Caroline put me to bed with a cup of tea and I fell into a feverish semi-coma. I still hadn't realised I had malaria, but the Mackies recognised the symptoms right away and Angus phoned his sister who was a doctor. She told them what to do and I had superb treatment, recovering after about three days. Fortunately, this was non-cerebral malaria, unlike my previous bout when I was hospitalised for two weeks.

Angus was also an ex-Army officer and our connection was a friendship with Spook Pittman, who had been in the QDG with me. After the army, he became a private pilot, eventually retiring to Zambia. The Mackies could not have been better hosts and also opened up their home when another good friend, Andrew Hartley, arrived. As mentioned before, Andrew always turns up in the most remarkable places, so although delighted to see him, I was hardly surprised. Once Millie and Thomasina arrived, we would all later meet up for a cruise down the Zambezi.

The main reason for the girls' trip was that Thomasina's father had recently died from Parkinson's-related causes and she was so taken by what I was doing that she contributed a significant amount of money towards the film being made of the odyssey. All of this was done via the crowdfunding website Indiegogo, and one of the incentive rewards was to travel with me for a section of the journey – which Thomasina won. The girls had organised an itinerary, and it would be a nice break for all of us.

Knowing Zambia well, Angus cast his eye over the itinerary and noted the girls had understandably not taken into account the size of Zambia and that consequently we would be spending most of our time driving around in a hired car, which would be costly and not interesting. He instead re-routed us to Livingstone to see the Victoria Falls and game reserves in the lower Zambezi valley and he even lent us his car.

What followed was a spectacular trip into the heart of Africa, with all the usual excitement of getting stuck in the sand, mechanical problems with fuel systems and punctures in the bush. Victoria Falls is rightly a World Heritage Site and the lower Zambezi is great for kayaking and seeing wild animals up close. Too close on one occasion, as when walking to our tent in the Kasaka River Lodge, an elephant trumpeted at us in the dark from barely ten yards away. I think I got more of a fright than the girls.

Millie and Thomasina left after two weeks, and I was sorry to see them go, as they had been great company and immaculate guests at the Mackies', making up for me being such a demanding git. They filmed a number of important pieces to camera as well, talking about being the daughters of fathers with Parkinson's.

While waiting for my Angolan visa, Angus and I went to the neurological hospital in Lusaka to interview people with Parkinson's – most importantly, Guy Scott.

He was a fascinating character, the only white person to be a president of any African country elected in a fully democratic election. It happened by default as Guy, a Zambian through and through, was vice-president when President Michael Sata died in 2014. He ruled as acting president for the next ninety days until a new election was held, as under that country's law no person without a direct Zambian bloodline can be president.

Now seventy-nine years old, he has advanced Parkinson's and is not easy to understand. But that does not stop him from courageously campaigning and speaking out about the disease. During our interview he told me that as an ex-farmer he firmly believed pesticides are the most prevalent cause of Parkinson's.

I also spoke to others living with the disease at Lusaka's teaching hospital. We spoke mainly about the high price and scarcity of Parkinson's medicines, and it was a sobering thought that these people were the lucky ones. Those outside the capital got no medical support at all.

I had one particularly moving conversation with a woman who hadn't told her family she had Parkinson's. They obviously knew something was wrong with her, but she tried her best to carry on living normally. I urged her to speak to them, saying she had nothing to worry about and they would understand. She phoned me the next day in tears, saying she had taken my advice and it was the best thing she'd done. Her family had pledged all the support she needed.

It was time to fly back to Angola and I couldn't thank Angus and Caroline enough for everything, not only for nursing me back to health but for their outstanding generosity. While it may never be possible to thank those who have helped me directly, I can follow their example and I go out of my way to be generous to others.

Back in Luanda, I got more welcome news. Another great friend from the QDG, Mark Ashley-Miller, was coming out to join me as he'd heard that I was having difficulty in driving myself. That was not quite true. I welcomed help, but I didn't need rescuing. However, Mark was having none of that. He was flying to Luanda within a couple of days, and we would spend the next two weeks driving down to Windhoek in Namibia.

I was certainly looking forward to it as Mark is not only tremendous fun, he would share a spectacular leg of the journey. Despite what I had been told, Angola was turning out to be one of the best countries I had yet visited.

34

Angola to Namibia

Mark arrived with the spare prop shaft spline and bearings – the fourth time Rob had shipped out motor spares in civilian hand luggage. Once again, no one in customs batted an eyelid and I jubilantly handed over the spare parts to Sammy, confident the wagon would soon be fixed.

My jubilation was short-lived. To my astonishment, the new parts didn't fit. I'm not sure what happened, as Rob is such an expert, but the trouble with Volkswagen's wide range of Transporter and California vans is that components that look exactly the same are not always interchangeable. Even with the chassis and engine numbers – which Rob practically knew by heart – it's sometimes difficult to pinpoint the exact spare part.

But it was not as serious as it first seemed and Sammy had a plan. If he took off the faulty prop shaft, the 4x4 van would revert to a standard two-wheel drive. As the worst of the roads were behind us and the monsoons were no longer a threat, we could probably reach Namibia on two-wheel drive. Namibia is a former German colony – albeit going back to the First World War – and there would be no shortage of Volkswagen garages. Sammy was already in contact with dealers there.

This would cause a bit of a delay, but if we had to hang around waiting for a vehicle to get fixed, we could do far worse than being stuck in Luanda. The restaurants were excellent and inexpensive, the hospitality at the British embassy superb and the city itself friendly and fascinating.

It also gave me the opportunity to do some Parkinson's awareness work. Being unable to speak Portuguese, it was more difficult for me to get TV networks interested than it had been in the francophone countries. However, I had an interview with National Radio Angola, which broadcasts in English on their international channel and although it only has a small audience, at least I was on air. It turned out to be one of the most fulfilling radio chats I've done. The interviewer totally related to my message and asked excellent questions – really getting to the crux of the major problems facing Parkinson's sufferers in Africa. After the interview we found ourselves talking about the consequences of colonialism and, to my surprise, he was very pro-British. Luanda had been a major slave-trading port in the eighteenth and nineteenth centuries, and as I'd found elsewhere in Africa, the abolition efforts of William Wilberforce and his mates as well as the work of the Royal Navy are given far more credit by descendants of slaves than most historians do in Britain.

It was now time to leave the capital and Mark and I first headed east to see the Kalandula Falls which, at 344 feet high and 1,300 feet wide, is one of the largest waterfalls by volume in Africa. Even in the dry season it was impressive. From there we headed south-west, hugging the coastline. The beaches were magnificent and I have some great photos of Mark and I wild camping at Binga Bay, a stunning cove with white sand, crystal waters and not another tourist in sight. It was perhaps the most beautiful spot I'd visited on the entire journey.

We then turned inland for Lubango, the country's second-largest city, as I needed to replace the wagon's tyres that had blistered from continuously banging into potholes over the past few months. The tyre shop was managed by Ruben Oliveira, who not only sourced what I wanted, but invited us to camp in his garden. He spoke reasonably good English, very unusual in that part of the world, and was keen to show us the positive side of his country. He stressed that the civil war that erupted after the Portuguese colonialists fled in 1974 had actually ended in 2002 and the country was now not only safe for tourists, but prospering.

He was absolutely right. Although we saw some burnt-out Soviet tanks, relics of the war fought by three internal liberation movements as well as Cuba and South Africa, it was patently clear that Angola was very much at peace with itself. I experienced that first-hand as everywhere we went – from the beaches to smoke-filled city restaurants and bars or just walking around town centres – we were warmly received.

With Ruben as our self-appointed guide, Mark and I went to places we would never have heard of, let alone seen. One such location was the Tundavala Gap, a huge, spectacular 7,390-foot fissure in the Serra da Leba Mountains overlooking a seemingly endless plateau; another was the 98-foot marble statue of Christ with outspread arms on a hill overlooking Lubango. It's a replica of the iconic Christ the Redeemer statue in Rio de Janeiro and one of only four in the world.

We could have carried on exploring this magnificent country, but time was tight and without a prop shaft I was wary about being too adventurous off-road. It was time to cross over into Namibia – which had been described to me as 'Africa for beginners'. It has great game reserves and wilderness, but is more orderly than many other fast-developing countries. In other words, no wild and woolly separatist movements, ubiquitous roadblocks and not-so-subtle demands for 'donations'.

First impressions confirmed this when Mark and I were efficiently ushered into the country at a well-swept and tidy border post by courteous officials. Surprisingly, English is the official language, even though it is the mother tongue of only three per cent of the population. Not only that, we were now driving on the 'correct' side of the road – for English people anyway.

The first town after the border was Ongwediva and, to my delight, I found the Volkswagen garage that Sammy had been talking to – the first I had come across in Africa. We pulled in to see if they could fix the prop shaft. It was strange being served by people in white shirts and ties and waiting in a comfortable leather armchair next to a coffee machine. I was used to bush mechanics like Sammy and Moses, people who could work wonders with little more than a spanner and spit and here was a fully equipped workshop with the most modern tools. Mark and I were by far the scruffiest people in the building but, despite that, the manager let us park on the forecourt and spend the night there.

Unfortunately, they couldn't fix the prop shaft, but after hearing about the Parkinson's odyssey from Mark – who was great at singing my praises – mechanics serviced the van for free.

Mark now had to fly back to the UK and got a lift to Windhoek airport with one of the garage's drivers, while I decided to remain in northern Namibia and wait for Rob Hayward to arrive. I needed a place to stay and, while driving on the main road, I saw a campsite sign with an arrow pointing down a dirt track. Not sure what to expect, I turned off and about two miles later arrived at a farmhouse. There to meet me was an extraordinary family – who did indeed run a campsite, charging a pittance to stay.

I soon realised I was in true hillbilly country straight out of *Deliverance*. The farm was owned by a former policeman, an avid big game hunter whose house was adorned with trophies of all sorts of animals. His equally aged wife never seemed to leave the kitchen. Their two sons who managed the business were tiny, almost dwarf-like, but built like blockhouses – as wide as they were tall. They both spoke with strange, falsetto voices, but were charming in an almost archaic way. The campsite was basic in the extreme, with a long-drop toilet and open-air shower heated by flaming brushwood. It certainly worked and I had the best, hottest shower of my entire African trip.

Rob arrived the next day to film the last leg of the journey and I told him he had to meet these people who seemed to be from another planet. He was not as eager as I was, but certainly savoured the rather unusual experience. All that was missing was a banjo and some cousins doing a stomping square dance. Conversation didn't exactly flow, but I listened fascinated as they described their simple rustic life, living largely off the land as their forefathers had done for well over a century.

From there we set off to the country's premier game reserve, the Etosha National Park, famed for having the largest salt pan in Africa. '*Etosha*' means 'white' in the local dialect, as the salt shimmers like a ghostly mirage in the arid countryside, and when the sparse summer rains fall, it's a magnet for wild animals. It's massive – 80 miles long and up to 31 miles wide – and visible from space.

It sounded good, but frankly I hated it. It was far too commercialised, with many hundreds of grey-haired tourists in pickup trucks and rooftop tents sipping gin and tonics while watching animals drinking on cue from floodlit waterholes. To me it was tantamount to a staged performance and I wanted no part of it. Forgetting for a moment that I too was a grey-haired tourist, I felt not only superior to these old couples enjoying their trip of a lifetime, but eager to get as much distance between us as possible.

With the wagon in two-wheel drive, we unfortunately couldn't travel along the much-vaunted Skeleton Coast – named for whale bones on the beaches and hundreds of ship wrecks. With a two-wheel drive, I discovered that Namibia was indeed Africa for beginners, and headed further down the coast, stopping at Walvis Bay, the country's main port and Swakopmund, a coastal resort with sandy beaches established by colonists in 1892. It was in that rather quaint Germanic town that I notched another first for me – a skydive.

Rob wanted to film this activity as an example of people afflicted with Parkinson's still being able to do things they never imagined they could. I was also keen, so we booked a parachute jump with Ground Rush Adventures, skydiving experts who were going to ensure I didn't plummet to the ground.

The view from several thousand feet in the air was beyond spectacular, with the Atlantic Ocean on one side and the Namib – the world's oldest desert – on the other. Linked in tandem to an instructor and freefalling at 125 m.p.h. we did all the spins and manoeuvres you can squeeze into thirty seconds before the parachute jolted open. Seven minutes later we floated to the ground.

Windhoek was directly inland and we headed east for the next four hours to one of the smallest and tidiest capital cities in Africa. Also unusual was that it had a superb campsite right in the heart of the city called Urban Camp, equipped with a beer garden, wifi, ATM, clean bathrooms and a sparkling pool surrounded by big shady trees.

Rob and I visited the country's main Volkswagen dealer in the rather forlorn hope of finding a spare prop shaft. Peter Barth, the manager shook his head – no such luck. I resigned myself to being limited to more sedate roads for the rest of the journey. It was a big blow.

Then that evening, long after other shops had closed, Peter phoned with an idea. Another customer with the same model vehicle as me was waiting for a new radiator to be shipped out from Germany. But the manager said if he could persuade the owner to trade his old prop shaft on condition that I bought him a new one that would be imported along with the radiator, we might have a solution.

I agreed on the spot, while the manager pointed out to the other bloke that he couldn't drive his vehicle while waiting for the radiator and would now get a brand-new prop shaft in the deal. I don't think I would ever have got such 'creative' service in the UK. The next day I had a fully operational 4x4 van again.

I enjoyed Windhoek immensely. Rob and I had the surreal experience of attending the annual beer festival that's based on the globally famous Munich Oktoberfest. I knew Namibia had a German legacy, but to see blonde Africans dressed in fake lederhosen and *fräuleins* in tight *dirndls* serving assembly-line steins of lager while bands blasted out oompah music was a sight to behold.

It was a great party – bettered only by the next evening when I was persuaded to accompany Lila Swanepoel, a filmmaker and Lee-Ray VIviers to a karaoke joint called Wolf Bar, where I was easily the oldest. I used to be able to sing quite well, but only in church or in private, but with unstoppable encouragement from Lila and Lee-Ray, I flicked through the available songs and chose 'American Pie' by Don McLean. Everyone knows it and it's a good singalong, but the DJ said it was too long for karaoke. I was about to quietly sneak back to my seat and half-drunk beer when I was told I could – no *should* – sing 'Bohemian Rhapsody' by Queen instead, which was longer and far more difficult. So if a Munich-style Oktoberfest in the middle of Africa was considered weird, that was nothing compared to a retired cavalry colonel emulating Freddie Mercury!

Namibia has a small population – about 2.5 million people – with a density of a mere eight people per square mile. Consequently, Parkinson's problems are not as prevalent as in the rest of Africa and, after interviewing one of the country's six neurologists, it seemed to me that the government had a reasonable handle on the disease.

Another great interview was with Sibongile 'Sibo' Tshabalala on a radio programme called *The Social*. During our chat, my phone started ringing, which would have been no real problem for anyone else, but for me to fish my mobile out from my pocket to turn it off quickly required a major feat of coordination. There was a bit of a pause, but Sibo handled it brilliantly, switching to the song 'Dancing on the Ceiling' by Lionel Richie, which I had said was my favourite. When she asked why I liked it, I replied that I wanted it played at my funeral as something cheerful while being carried out of the church in a coffin. She enjoyed that.

Next stop was Lüderitz, a beautiful little town far down the coast with a dark history. The nearby peninsula of Shark Island was used as a concentration camp by the Germans during the Namaqua and Herero uprisings. It's estimated up to three thousand indigenous people died in that camp between 1905–7.

After filming the sun setting behind the Shark Island lighthouse, we nearly had a disaster. Everybody knows that driving on gravel affords little grip, but perhaps I'd let my guard down as we travelled back to the town. While taking a corner a gentle slip turned into a slide, then a skid and, before I knew it, I was heading sideways for the edge of the road and a steep drop. We weren't going fast, but I realised that if I tried to correct the skid, I would risk flipping the wagon. Making a split-second decision, I deliberately steered straight into the bush, where after a series of ominous 'bangs' we came to a shuddering stop. But I had saved the vehicle, and probably us, from potential catastrophe.

The damage was significant but fixable. That's my motto in emergencies – if you're alive, everything is fixable. I had punctured one tyre, bent two wheel rims and also damaged the suspension – yet again!

It was now dark, and after two hours of hard work under torchlight, we managed to get the wagon mobile and drive the short distance back to Lüderitz. The local mechanic was a German-African called, if my memory serves me right, Walter Schmidt. His grandfather had set up the garage in the 1930s and steam tools in pristine condition were still in operation. He was brilliant, fixing the suspension problem in no time at all.

From Lüderitz, it was just a short hop to the South African border.

35

End of the Odyssey

The border between Namibia and South Africa is the Orange River. It's the longest river in southern Africa, rising 1,551 miles east in the tiny mountain kingdom of Lesotho and, as it nears the Atlantic, its gravel beds are rich with diamonds. Consequently, I expected something a little more impressive. Instead, I barely noticed we had crossed it.

However, I certainly noticed we were now in South Africa. It was ostentatiously another country, more modern than anywhere else on the continent. The roads down the Cape West Coast were good and we were tempted to stop off and see some of the beach towns. I then asked myself what I would do if I were travelling alone and the answer was simple: go directly to Cape Town and complete the mission.

The next day we arrived in what South Africans call the 'Mother City'. The country has three capitals: Pretoria, the administrative; Cape Town, the legislative and Bloemfontein, the judicial. But Cape Town is where the story of modern South Africa started and where my odyssey finished.

Rob had booked into a hotel, but I decided to camp as I have a thing about staying in plush places when there's a perfectly good van to sleep in. I dropped him off, then went to a campsite at the Strand, a seaside resort on the eastern perimeter of the city.

I'm glad I did. Even though Rob and I got on well, I desperately needed a couple of days on my own to decompress. I was exhausted. I had not eaten or slept well for months, was carrying the expectations of a significant number of well-wishers and sponsors on my shoulders and, despite medication, still had the daily grind of Parkinson's to contend with. I should have been elated, knocking back the champagne.

It was the opposite. I have never felt so deflated. I turned off the ignition and rested my head on the steering wheel, nearly in tears and did nothing. A journey that had been a dream for forty years and taken more than three to complete... was suddenly over.

Just like that.

I had been running on empty for so long that I was now well and truly finished. Although satisfied that the job was done, I felt far from triumphant. In fact, I felt more like a spent mayfly.

The Strand campsite was just across the road from the beach, and for the next two days I did nothing but chill out while I topped up my tanks. At the same time, Rob, the consummate filmmaker, worked hard in his hotel putting the documentary together.

Although the second stage of the odyssey had been billed as Freetown to Cape Town, I hadn't realised that Cape Town is not the southernmost tip of Africa. That honour belongs to Cape Agulhas, 140 miles further down, where the Indian and Atlantic oceans meet.

Once I'd recovered, Rob and I set off to film me at the edge of the continent. It's a spectacular drive over Sir Lowry's Pass, across the Hottentots Holland Mountain, and no one else was at the rocky Agulhas headland when we drove onto the pebble beach. For a brief moment, I was the most southerly person in Africa. It was then that it truly sank in that I was also probably the only person afflicted with Parkinson's to have traversed the entire continent by vehicle. I put my hand on the wagon and said, 'Thank you.'

I afforded myself a congratulatory pat on the back. I had received a number of accolades and comments of support and respect for what I was doing, but up until then I did not appreciate them. Now, at last, I did.

One thing I had to get used to in South Africa was the security situation, a legacy of the apartheid era which legalised discrimination against the indigenous black people. I had spent much of the past eight months sleeping on the side of the road either in the bush or in cities, often buying food at ramshackle kiosks in shanty towns, rubbing shoulders with street people and never felt seriously threatened. In South Africa, officially ranked as one of the most violent countries in the world, it's different. Although most places in central Cape Town itself are safe to walk around in during the day, everyone in the wealthier areas lives either in gated communities or behind high walls and razor wire. There was no question of me sleeping rough.

Consequently, I moved in with Luigi Watterson and his wife at the foot of Table Mountain for the next week. Luigi had left the Queen's Dragoon Guards soon after I joined and, although I had not seen him in thirty-five years, the regimental bond is so strong that any member is a comrade for life. I spent most of my stay patching up the van for it to be shipped back to the UK, but also did tourist stuff like going up Table Mountain, one of southern Africa's most iconic landmarks.

My mission now completed, I no longer needed the support of the British embassy, although I was invited to a lunch party by the defence attaché. To my amazement I met my Sandhurst platoon commander at the lunch. Chris Vernon had set me off on my military journey nearly four decades ago and this seemed to be a fitting reunion. I thought of another coincidence: James Moberly – one of my best friends at Durham University – had also been in Chris Vernon's platoon and had started the odyssey with me in France. I was now ending it where James's father had once been stationed: Sir Patrick Moberly had been Britain's ambassador to South Africa in the 1980s.

I was still keen to spread the Parkinson's awareness message and was interviewed by Rodney Trudgeon on Fine Music Radio, which bills itself as Africa's only classical and jazz radio station. The programme was *People of Note*, in British terms a mixture of Classic FM and *Desert Island Discs*. I was asked to name my favourite five records, but as choices were limited to classical music, that proved to be a bit difficult. It was the only radio interview I did in South Africa, yet was one of the most enjoyable I'd done on my journey.

The key South African interview for the odyssey documentary was with Professor Jonathan Carr who, as head of the Division of Neurology at Tygerberg hospital, is the leading neurosurgeon teaching in Africa. He was charming and eloquent, but while I was hoping for an upbeat message to cap the journey he was brutally honest, saying he doubted we would see a cure in my lifetime. On the plus side, he said, 'immense effort, energy and money' were being spent on research. 'The unbelievable work by the Michael J. Fox Foundation has placed colossal emphasis on making a difference to patients in terms of therapy. So I think there is some optimism at the immense scientific energy spent on this [Parkinson's] and similar conditions, and helping one is likely to help all,' he said. 'Alzheimer's is the commoner disease, but has a lot of similarities to Parkinson's. So a potential cure for Alzheimer's might open the door for other similar conditions. But it's a waiting game.'

He agreed with me that in Africa, awareness was one of the most fundamental issues. 'Small investments will make a colossal difference to knowing what Parkinson's actually is. Although the current median age in Africa is eighteen, the population is ageing and there will be a growing need of Parkinson's awareness in the future. We need to alleviate people of uncertainty by providing simple information.'

That, in a nutshell, is what my voyage was all about.

The African odyssey itself was over and what I now wanted to do was to visit a battleground etched into the psyche of every

British military person: Rorke's Drift. In fact, 'visit' is too soft a word. I wanted to pay homage to one of the most heroic clashes in British military history; a desperate battle fought with whatever weapons were available – rifles, pistols, assegais – a spear used mostly in southern Africa – bayonets, clubs, knives and fists. Eleven men of the 24th Regiment of Foot won Victoria Crosses that day, the most ever received for a single action by one regiment.

I flew to Durban and hired a car, heading north towards the Tugela River, the border – both physical and spiritual – of Zululand. This was the other face of South Africa, wild and rugged, the flipside of Cape Town's shopping malls and Michelin-star restaurants. Everything in deep Zululand was different; the dilapidated *spaza* shops selling basic goods, dusty roads, scrawny goats and mud and thatch huts. As there was no mobile signal, I was navigating by compass and not sure exactly where I was.

Suddenly a car stopped in front and three young black men got out. I had been warned about this – hijacking and brutal assaults were common in the dodgier areas – so I braced myself. Even so, I felt strangely at ease, as if I knew I was in no danger. They came up to my window and motioned me to wind it down. 'Where are you going?' one asked.

'To the lodge at Rorke's Drift.'

He looked at me for a moment. 'There is no lodge at Rorke's Drift, but there is one further along on this road. Follow us.'

I was aware that few white South Africans would have opened their window and almost certainly would have accelerated off the moment the three men appeared. But I still felt confident they meant me no harm. Or perhaps, I was being incredibly naïve. They could have been leading me anywhere. Anyway, I followed the car a fair distance and eventually up a long driveway with a large house at the end. One of the men got out and gestured that I should come with him. He rang the doorbell. A white man opened the door, asking what we wanted.

With a brief wave, the three black men drove off. Just another act of extraordinary kindness by random strangers – made even more moving in a crime-riddled country.

'I'm looking for a room for the night,' I said to the man, whom I presumed to be the lodge manager.

'Sorry, we're closed. We're shut for the entire winter to do renovations.' I had no idea what to do next. All I knew was that I was in potential trouble, stuck in the bush at night, not really knowing where I was. The innkeeper, whose name was Shane, sensed this and relented. 'OK, come in. I'll make a bed for you.'

It was incredibly generous as he had to open up the entire hotel to make just one bed. Not only that, his wife cooked me a meal. They were interested in my story and also organised a guide to take me to the battlefields the next day.

The guide, an ex-policeman who had lost a leg, drove me first to Isandlwana, where in 1879 the British Army suffered one of its worst defeats against an indigenous foe equipped with vastly inferior weapons. My guide drove me up a hill with a panoramic view of the battlefield. It was an eerie experience seeing the veld strewn with white-painted stones that marked the exact spots where each of the more than 1,300 British and colonial soldiers had fallen, including my wife's great-great-great uncle, Lieutenant George Hodson of the 1st Battalion, 24th Regiment of Foot. I spent the morning there, mesmerised by the profound historical aura, and in the afternoon we went to Rorke's Drift. As mentioned, for me and most British soldiers, this was truly hallowed ground. However, my guide was dismissive of the importance of the battle, saying it was more of a Zulu cattle raid on a minor outpost than a military offensive. If the Zulus had attacked with a force of four thousand warriors, as some history books claim, my guide was adamant that the 139-strong British garrison simply would not have had enough ammunition to repel them.

Be that as it may, no one disputes that the British soldiers, some lame and sick, fought for their lives with unbelievable heroism.

The battle itself is deservedly famous, but what is not that well-known are the sad consequences for some of the Victoria Cross recipients. Private Robert Jones, who was repeatedly engaged in hand-to-hand fighting, later committed suicide; William Jones had to pawn his medal to put food on the table and was buried in a pauper's grave, while Christian Schiess became a beggar on the streets of Cape Town. When the Royal Navy found him five years later, suffering from dreadful exposure and malnutrition, he was put on a ship to Britain. He died en route and was buried at sea. He was just twenty-eight.

In fact, five of the eleven recipients, including the commanders Colonel John Chard and Lieutenant Gonville Bromhead, died before the age of fifty. Times have changed, and today we are better at looking after our soldiers – but still not good enough. We need to try even harder on their behalf.

The next day I went to Spion Kop, another battle where Britain got a bloody nose, this time at the hands of the Boers. The irony was that Britain should have won, as we had pushed the Boers off the Spion Kop hill, but after the commander, Major-General Edward Woodgate, was killed, a confused order was given to withdraw. The Lancashire Fusiliers consequently suffered a huge loss, with two hundred soldiers killed, and their remains still lie on the hill in a mass grave. But the name lives on as 'the Kop', one of the stands at Liverpool Football Club's home Anfield Stadium, which serves as an everlasting memorial to those who paid the ultimate price.

Both Winston Churchill and Mahatma Gandhi, the latter a stretcher-bearer for the British, were present at that battle. It's also engraved in my memory from school history lessons – and as the mass grave attests, Kipling's poem 'Tommy Atkins' on the debt we as a nation owe to the ordinary British soldier is poignantly stark.

I flew back to the Cape and stayed in Stellenbosch with Lucy Erskine, a family friend, while I sorted out the last chore of the odyssey: to get the valiant wagon home. I phoned Duncan

Johnson of African Overlanders – a veteran Africa traveller himself, albeit on motorbikes – who specialises in shipping and asked what needed to be done. 'Just bring the van to my yard when you're about to leave,' he said, 'and we'll do the rest.'

'Is that all? What about the paperwork?'

'Just leave it with me.'

I was a little suspicious. Surely it couldn't be that easy? 'When will it arrive in the UK?' I asked.

'I'll let you know when it's on the water and it'll arrive three weeks after that. I just need to find a container to share with another vehicle.'

He quoted me a price, which turned out to be cheaper than I later paid moving house a single mile from one village to the next in Dorset. It all seemed too good to be true, but on my last day, I drove to his farm, parked the wagon among several other overland vehicles and handed him the keys.

We went to town for a pizza and beer, then I caught a taxi to the airport.

The next day I was home.

36

Hannington

With only hand luggage – everything else was stored in the wagon – I caught the late train from London to Sherborne, where I was met by Mark Ashley-Miller. As we jumped into his car, I ruefully remarked that we were a long way from Angola.

His smile said it all: 'Welcome back.'

Waking up in my own bed the next morning after nine months on the road was a strange sensation, as well as a time for reflection. While happy that I had achieved my goal, the reality is that Parkinson's does not have a happy ending. There are no winners. You have to make the most of every moment, as every day sees the pendulum swinging between OK moments and bad moments with the occasional good moment thrown in. And I had to face the reality that I probably wouldn't be able to do such a gruelling trip again. As any overlander will attest, travelling in Africa is an exhausting test of endurance and grit mixed with sheer exuberance like none other. When you're on a Parkinson's plummet, it's obviously even more challenging.

The main thing that struck me now the voyage was over was that having a daily sense of purpose was one of the best ways to cope with this wretched affliction. While travelling, I was continuously dealing with situations, some of my own making, others out of my control. But whatever the problem was, it was up to me to fix it. Although Parkinson's was always ticking ominously in the background, it rarely was the core issue as I had other challenges to overcome. No matter how knackered or incapable, I had no choice but to get on with the job in hand. There was no alternative.

Back in England, I no longer had an overriding sense of purpose to occupy me. Without that, the disease slithers back into your mind and body like a repellent monster.

I realised I had to have something to live for. Something to get me up in the morning. That is something I tell myself every day and I urge other people with Parkinson's to do the same. For me that 'something' was fast coalescing as a desire to try my best to assist others also afflicted. But first of all I had to capitalise on the journey I had just made – write it up, publicise it, show the film and use it as a platform to tell my story.

A couple of weeks later I got a message from the Cape Town shipper, Duncan Johnson, telling me which day the wagon would be arriving at Tilbury docks.

I was still vaguely suspicious about how ridiculously simple it seemed, but sure enough, on the given date, the ship arrived. Wilfred was with me and – once we had ploughed our way through acres of containers piled to the sky and found the wagon – all I had to do was sign for it and pump up one of the tyres. It had been a faithful companion and servant – my home in which I'd cried, laughed, spent time with friends and seen wonderful parts of the world. It's now with me in Dorset; mission accomplished.

Perhaps the most useful 'skill' required for travelling in Africa – or anywhere – was one I have tried to exercise ever since joining the Army. It's simply this: treat all people as you would wish to be treated yourself. As decent human beings. Nothing more, nothing less. Sharing a cigarette while cooped up in a tank with three rough and ready troopers from the other side of the street was a great leveller and there was no better way of knowing what was *really* going on in the squadron. Consequently, as an officer – a 'Rupert' as our men called us when out of earshot – I went out of my way to talk to the common soldier. It was not something I felt I had to do; I did it because I genuinely liked most of them. It was no big deal, but to my eternal gratitude, I found that the respect and camaraderie I showed was repaid to a degree I did not deserve.

It was exactly the same in Africa. When stranded on the side of the street, I found that time and time again people helped me purely out of the kindness of their hearts. I always acknowledged that, showing my genuine appreciation and, as my story tells, they almost always not only responded, but went the extra mile. Despite the language gaps, I found ordinary folk throughout the continent incredibly easy to talk to, happy despite their often difficult circumstances and demanding nothing in return for giving me a hand. I instinctively reciprocated that eagerness to communicate, whether bumping along potholed roads listening to blaring music with hardy truck drivers in Angola or savouring a chocolate sandwich on a desert track in Mauritania.

Africa showed me that there is far more good than bad in this world – and even bad people are not bad all the time. As long as you have a relationship with them, you will get on. I'm comfortably off by England's standards, but in most of Africa I was a millionaire, travelling across their continent in an expensive vehicle loaded with fancy equipment, cameras and radios. Yet only once or twice was anything stolen and it was entirely my own fault. By and large, people were respectful of what was mine, despite their often abject poverty.

However, above all, I learned about the unyielding heroism of so many people living with Parkinson's, people who have done far more than I have and shown so much courage. Just thinking of the spectacular work Hilaire Roger does in Cameroon with little or no help shames me to my core whenever I complain. Consequently, I have vowed that when I talk about Parkinson's, it's not about me – it's about people who have a far more horrible time than I or any sufferer in the west can even imagine. However miserable I feel at times, many millions of others have it far worse.

Which brings me to Hannington Kabugo, one of the most remarkable men I've ever met.

I had been told about Hannington by the Parkinson's Africa organisation and as he lives in Uganda, some way off my route, I interviewed him on Zoom while I was in Namibia. It was not a satisfactory discussion and I promised I would fly out to Kampala and meet him personally once the odyssey was completed.

Seven months later, I kept that promise. Hannington was there to meet me at the airport and show me first-hand the work he did. His story is enough to make the angels weep.

When Hannington was fifteen, his mother Milly's health deteriorated alarmingly. She shook continuously, her speech was slurred, she kept falling over and had constant anxiety attacks. Hannington's father called in a witchdoctor. His diagnosis was predictable: she had been cursed and the family must leave her or else they would suffer the same fate. As a result, Milly was locked inside the house and the family went to live elsewhere so her 'evilness' could not spread. Mr Kabugo instructed his children they must never see their mother again. They obeyed.

Except Hannington. He went back to visit his mother on weekends. He spoke to her through the window. In tears, she begged him to leave as she thought the 'curse' was contagious. Hannington refused, arriving to see her the next weekend. And the next. He never stopped. 'I loved her so much,' he told me. Milly survived on one meagre meal a day, pushed under the door with a long pole by a good Samaritan neighbour. 'That woman was my mother's angel,' said Hannington.

Indeed.

Everyone in the area was poor and not always able to feed themselves adequately, much less their neighbours, and on one occasion, Hannington arrived to find that Milly hadn't been fed for several days. He looked through the window. She was lying on the floor, curled in a foetal position. Hannington could see scratch marks where she had scraped mud off the earthen floor to eat.

Every day, in pain and depression so deep it's impossible to fathom, Milly prayed that she would die. After five years her wish was granted, but in the saddest way possible. She died alone, wracked with tremors and utter misery. Her body was discovered several days later.

Hannington vowed to do something about what his mother had been through and scoured the internet, searching for sicknesses that involved uncontrollable shakes. Thanks to Google, he came across a disease called Parkinson's. Milly had all the symptoms – falling, slurred speech, tremors – it was a classic case. He kept googling and discovered Parkinson's is not transferable or contagious. It's a straightforward neurological condition affecting millions of people around the world. It was not a curse. His family had abandoned a loving wife and mother to an indescribable hell through sheer ignorance and on instructions from a witchdoctor.

At the time, Hannington worked as a civil servant earning about three hundred dollars a month. He used his money to print posters stating a simple message: '*Parkinson's Si Buko*' ('Parkinson's Is Not Witchcraft'), illustrated with photos of bent white people walking with sticks, as he couldn't find pictures of black sufferers on the internet. He outlined the symptoms and urged people to phone him if they or someone they knew suffered from the disease. He then asked taxi drivers if he could put the posters up on their minibuses and several agreed.

Hannington's phone started ringing the next day. And the next. People were calling in saying, 'I think my father has this.' Or an aunt. An uncle. A brother.

With a few simple stickers and the goodwill of a few taxi drivers, Hannington became a lightning rod for Parkinson's disease in Uganda. His phone rang daily. He kept a register of callers and hired a village hall for a meeting, paying for it with his own meagre earnings. The small venue was jammed with about a hundred people.

'This is not your fault,' Hannington repeatedly told them. 'You are not cursed.'

None of the sufferers or those helping them had heard about Parkinson's. None of them knew what was afflicting them. With a shock, Hannington realised he was the only person in the room aware of what Parkinson's actually was: a straightforward neurological condition. They all thought they were cursed. He organised another conference, but this time he hired – again out of his own pocket – one of Uganda's few neurologists to speak. It was the first time these people had heard a doctor tell them what was wrong with them. And that they were not cursed.

From there, Hannington ran awareness programmes showing people what symptoms to look for and teaching health carers at grassroots clinics to recognise the disease. Previously, many Ugandan doctors misdiagnosed Parkinson's as a stroke or alcohol abuse – even when patients had never drunk due to religious beliefs. He got the more seriously ill to clinics and urged families of those who couldn't afford medication – in other words, the overwhelming majority – to show the love and acceptance which sufferers needed more than anything else. A hug went a long way, he stressed, as Parkinson's wasn't contagious.

'Don't lock them away in a hut and leave them,' he said again and again.

Slowly, through unshakeable grit and enormous energy, he has almost singlehandedly dispelled the stigma surrounding the disease in at least four areas of Uganda. His achievement is simply staggering, as in rural Africa merely eradicating the stigma is as big a deal as finding an actual cure.

He did that using his own money, so I'm setting up a charity that will be able to help him – and others, like Hilaire – in their work. All royalties from this book and the documentary Rob and I made will go to Parkinson's charities, including a fund which will support people like Hannington who do so much with so little. Obviously, the main thrust is to find a cure, but there are numerous other expenses, such as paying taxi fares for Parkinson's sufferers to get to hospitals, hiring village halls to spread awareness messages, financing the printing costs of posters and conducting censuses of Parkinson's sufferers. Once the numbers are known, pressure can be brought on governments to get medicines and train neurologists. I know it's just one more problem, like malaria or Ebola, which are even more pressing, but as the population ages in Africa, Parkinson's is going to become increasingly prevalent. As it does not kill, the burden of care is going to be an immense challenge to communities that already have enough to worry about.

Hannington showed the way forward. Even if we don't find a cure soon, we can still change people's lives by helping them understand what they are going through – that it's not their fault and that they are normal people. That alone can make life worthwhile and spare those with the condition the dreadful misery Hannington's mother faced as she prayed for death. To this day, every time Hannington speaks of her, tears stream down his face.

But there's one thing I'm certain of: Milly Kabugo is up there somewhere, cured and at peace, looking down on her extraordinary son with absolute pride.

I may not have known it when I first set out on my African odyssey, but Hannington's story is the essence of what the trip was about. It started as a dream, but ended up as so much more. For I have seen first-hand people fighting the medical equivalent of Rorke's Drift every moment of their lives without medicine, without hospital care, without help and without expectation. Yet still they do not give up.

Not only that, I am sure there are many more people like Hannington, Hilaire, Omotola and the good Samaritan who pushed food under Milly Kabugo's door whom we don't know about. Good people still out there in Africa's remote areas, feeding and caring for those living in unspeakable desolation who need our help. It is for them that I wrote this book and it will be they who will be the ultimate beneficiaries from any profit. This will be through the Deacon Foundation, which aims to support those engaged in the battle against Parkinson's at the lowest level: the true frontline.

As I said, with Parkinson's there is no happy ending and I must be realistic. I should probably accept that a return journey from South Africa up the East Coast of Africa may be too much for me. Although it would be easier than travelling down the West Coast and I have learned many lessons, I may never be able to do such a demanding trip through Africa again and as each day passes, Parkinson's adds another straw to the pile making such a journey less likely.

However, that does not mean I'm giving up. I have three other potential voyages on the drawing board; one circumnavigating the Black Sea coastline, another around the shores of the Baltic Sea and the third through the Balkans. The Black Sea is on hold as at the time of writing the Russia–Ukraine war still rages, but the others are very much on my mind if Africa is too much for me.

I might not be able to do them all alone, as every year the ravages of Parkinson's exponentially undermine my abilities. But the message will be the same: don't sit around waiting to die; the men at Rorke's Drift didn't.

That's not for me – and I hope not for you.

Acknowledgements

So many people stand out for helping me on this journey. I simply could not have done it by myself. What follows is more or less in chronological order but not quite. Inevitably, I will not remember everything about everybody. Please forgive me. There are names I did not keep or did not catch at the time and some listed below get only six words when, in fact, they showed such extraordinary kindness that they deserve a chapter.

Alex Beeley, for persuading me to stick to my aspirations when I doubted them.

Andrew and Sue Spink, for being ever supportive and helpful in every possible way. They still are.

Scott Robinson, for helping me with the initial practical jobs that needed doing to prepare the van.

Charlie le Poidevin, for keeping me sane and on track when packing to leave.

Nick Woolgar, for acting as my backstop and clearing up loose ends on my departure.

Wareham Quay fabricators, for building VW accessories to my own design.

Breeze Commercial Vehicles, for servicing the wagon prior to departure and on return.

Rob Willis @ Volkstrek, for preparing the wagon for the adventure ahead and remaining ever available to help resolve every mechanical issue I had along the way. And for literally going the extra mile to make sure I had the right spare parts available to me.

James Moberly, for joining me for the opening weeks of the journey through France and for being a constant supporter for forty-two years.

Andrew Hartley, for providing inspiration in 1981 and for being the driving force behind the Deacon Foundation.

Chris Forrest, for providing advice and encouragement, lending me equipment, providing accommodation in France and always being available.

Mohammed, for working overtime and with good humour to fix my differential in Andorra and not killing me with my reintroduction to medicinal marijuana. And for extraordinary hospitality in Morocco.

Jimmy Thomas, for being excellent company and help when stranded in Andorra.

Christina Hippisley, for bringing out essential equipment to Portugal.

Frank McClintock, for accommodating me in Portugal.

Sue le Poidevin, for letting me stay while in Portugal, helping black out the windows and providing the mattress on which I spent the next many months sleeping. And for not being shocked by Anne Hathaway's portrayal of Maggie in *Love and Other Drugs*.

Emma and Alistair Bryant, for taking me into their family when in Rabat.

David Attenburrow, for joining me for two weeks and encouraging me to go where I might not have gone by myself or with others. For not being bored by technical discussions and understanding my motivation.

Jon Felton, for having me to stay in Laayoune and recognising that I needed to rest and recover.

Omar, for shaking off the troublesome fixer, for having me to stay and providing interesting memories.

Victor Ndiaye, for having me to stay for a very long time in Dakar, arranging my visas for Guinea and Guinea-Bissau and taking me into his family.

Tattie and Miriam, for showing me Dakar and laughing all the time.

Alain Monteiro, for servicing the wagon for nothing and being a thorough bloke.

Kamal and Mandi, for taking me in while I was in The Gambia.

John Harper, for dealing with my enquiries in the absence of a DA in Freetown and seeing me right on arrival.

Nick and Kim Gardner, for convincing me that Covid was serious and helping me make my plans. And for showing me around Freetown.

Martin Bamin, for taking me in when I first outstayed my welcome at the British complex in Freetown and on my return for being ever available and ultimately holding my farewell press/thank-you party at Mango Peak.

Jane and Matt Palmer, for putting me up in their house when they were in the process of moving out.

Jenny and Martin Travers. Well, it would have been impossible without their support, both in accommodating me when waiting for flights back to the UK while Covid was prevalent, looking after the wagon while I was back in the UK and accommodating me on my return while they were packing up to return to the UK.

Rob Hayward. More than can be stated. My longest accompanist, the owner of the plan to make a film, the maker of the film and for his consistent good humour.

Phoebe Vickers, for her great help in raising funds and overseeing my administration.

Nick Macleod-Ash, for early encouragement and access to technical support.

Gil Baldwin, for unfailing support and encouragement and for providing an introduction and proposing to Simplyhealth that they become my main sponsor.

Sneh Khemka, Chrissy Fice and Charlotte Cook at Simplyhealth, for being my main sponsor.

Teddy Wakefield, for responding instantly to my request for assistance and through MoyaApp and Data Free becoming my second sponsor.

Mark O'Reilly, owner of Mabway, one of my major sponsors.

Omotola Thomas, for establishing Parkinson's Africa and providing essential access in Africa, encouragement during the journey and deep support throughout the project.

Adrian Pennink, for offering essential advice on the production and promotion of the documentary.

Lisa Chesney, for personal interest and commitment and leading the staff of the British high commission in Freetown in their extraordinary support of the project.

Lieutenant Colonel Rob Browne, defence attaché, Freetown, for general support and returning unwanted equipment to the UK.

Solomon, for two years of care and devotion to the security and safekeeping of the wagon during the Covid lockdown.

Duncan Bullivant, for placing the support of Henderson's behind me to provide security and advice throughout the journey.

Ian Currie, for providing accommodation, advice and support, including cooking many meals during my stay in Monrovia.

Henry Joynson, for providing accommodation, advice, and support during my stay in Monrovia.

Sampson and Rufus, two individuals who spotted the wagon during the journey and introduced themselves to me, thus demonstrating that my message was getting out, and saying they wanted to help with Parkinson's.

Neil Bradley, for personal interest and commitment and leading the staff of the British high commission in Monrovia.

The Cameroonian diplomat who introduced me to her brother who is coping with Parkinson's with no medical support, just a loving family.

Albéric and Christaline de Colnet, for rescuing me from the side of the road in Côte d'Ivoire, having me to stay in Abidjan and helping get me out of deep trouble.

Papi and Johan, for tireless efforts to find solutions to the mechanical issues in Abidjan, for their interest in my mission and for committing the staff of the garage to fixing the wagon at a fraction of the cost price.

Hank Jansen, for giving up a week to deliver spare parts for the wagon, but, above all, for offering exactly the right support when I needed it most.

Chloe Grant, for providing excellent advice to all overland travellers via the West African Travellers WhatsApp group and providing me with refuge and assistance for the most difficult episode of the journey.

Dougie and Clara Young, for giving me access to their flat while marooned in Abidjan.

Thierry Gouegnon, for fixing my most effective media appearances.

Dan Frimpong, for supporting my application to enter Ghana and acting as my guarantor.

Sly, for driving me to Kumasi when I was incapable of driving alone.

Vida Obese, for arranging access to people with Parkinson's in Kumasi.

Harriet Thompson, British high commissioner, who solved the Nigeria visa issue.

Nick Hales, for accommodating me and helping me cross Togo and Benin.

Tim Hepworth, for doing *everything* for me and the cause during my time in Nigeria. And being very good company.

Tim Illingworth, for providing security, advice and company for my journey through Nigeria.

Julius, for seeing me safely across the border from Nigeria to Cameroon.

Abu, for driving me across the border to Cameroon.

Morin Desalu, for her total commitment to sufferers from Parkinson's in Nigeria and for arranging access to the press.

Keizey, for displaying a level of support and compassion beyond that of most, having never met me before.

Manga Bessem, Cameroon's ambassador in Yaoundé, for allowing me to enter Cameroon.

Lieutenant Odenoue, gendarme, who waited for me when I was late in arriving in Banyo.

The Cameroonian truck driver who bent every rule and transported me to Yaoundé with great humour.

Christian Dennys-McClure and Nigel Holmes, UK high commissioner and deputy, plus staff and the military mission, for accommodating me and shipping spare parts, administering and advising me, and Mireille for gaining excellent access to the press while in Cameroon.

Hilaire Roger, for the outstanding support he and his family give to people with Parkinson's and encouragement which continues to this day.

Roadside good Samaritans, Gloria, Kevin and Ben – the three travellers who stopped for me and got me going again on the road to Libreville, then stayed with me to make sure I was all right.

Piero, the outstanding bush mechanic in Lalara.

Ali, fellow traveller, the chap who shared a ride with me from Lalara and ensured I made it safely to the hotel where I was to meet Rob.

Marcel, for arranging our activities in Gabon, fixing visas and gaining access to filming subjects in Gabon.

Jannie Fourie, for keeping me optimistic and level-headed when I was at the end of my tether and providing a change of scene when most needed.

Moses, the best bush mechanic I came across on the entire trip.

Wilfred Deacon, for enduring me at my least impressive and seeing me safely to the Congo border.

Elle Rickett, for driving around the UK late into the night in search of spare parts.

The Dolisie garage attendant, whose name I didn't catch, who offered me the staff facilities and organised her brother to drive me to Pointe-Noire.

Jofran, that brother, for driving me to Pointe-Noire and ensuring I was safely accommodated, for finding backstreet mechanics and for his love of the music of the *Pipes and Drums of the Scots Guards*, which we played solidly for the four-hour journey.

Damian, for company and advice plus research into the various routes from Pointe-Noire to Matadi.

Pascal, Pointe-Noire restaurateur, for letting me set up camp in his car park on the beach.

Roger Stringer and the staff of the Angolan embassy, for not having a fit when I arrived against his instructions on the back of an eighteen-wheeler, for providing accommodation, meals and being excellent company.

Sammy, for getting the wagon back into a state in which it could carry on the journey.

Angus and Caroline Mackie, for everything. There are not enough superlatives to describe how kind the Mackies were. From nursing me through malaria to knowing when to ignore me and from acting as travel agents to film-camera operators, I am left eternally indebted to this couple.

The good Samaritan at the airport in Lusaka, for helping me off the aircraft when I was at my weakest.

Thomasina Bowyer-Bower, for being the single most generous sponsor and joining me and Millie in Zambia, where she was such good company.

Millie Deacon, for coping with her father in his hours of weakness and, with Thomasina, explaining to all on film what it is like to have a parent with a chronic illness.

Mark Ashley-Miller, for making the Angola leg of my trip truly memorable and for consistent support from home.

Luigi Watterson, for assisting in seeking spare parts and accommodating me in Cape Town.

Ruben Oliveira, for providing a place to camp and showing me Lubango and the real Angola.

Keizy of VW Ondangwa, for providing accommodation and servicing the wagon in Namibia.

All VW outlets in Namibia. Without exception all VW employees were as helpful as it was possible to be, with every single creak and knock investigated and more inspections than the wagon had had in the previous ten years.

Chrissy @ Overland Campers, for being an excellent hostess in Windhoek. And running one of the best campsites I stayed in.

Lila Swanepoel and Lee-Ray VIviers, for showing me the delights of Windhoek.

Peter Barth, VW Windhoek, for finally finding a solution to the prop shaft problem.

Lucy Erskine, for having me to stay in Stellenbosch.

Duncan Johnson, for shipping the vehicle back to the UK.

Ben Spink, for building the website.

Nick Fox, for seizing the project and marketing the film and the book.

Victoria Lyne-Pirkis, for finding a publisher and for publicising the project.

Hannington Kabugo, for showing us his excellent work in Uganda and setting the standard in raising awareness in Africa.

Ian Macfarlane-Bowman, for creating the Deacon Foundation.

All those who have offered venues for presentations.

Graham Spence, for extracting a story from my notes, diary and dictation.

Roland Ladley, for having the vision to see a tale that others might be interested in.

Helen Matthews and all at Cure Parkinson's, both for their support for the project and driving the search for a cure.

The 253 donors who responded to the call to fund the film.

And a further thank-you to all those who followed me on Polarsteps as I headed south. Knowing that I had a number of followers who were genuinely interested in what I was doing was extremely motivating. Without the knowledge that there were people all over the world wishing me well and offering encouragement I could, in my darker moments, have given the whole thing up, accepted I was the wrong side of sixty and settled down to a life of obscurity, waiting for time to pass. Thanks to all those people, I did not, and I will not.

And of course, to Tania, who has supported me in every way for the last twenty-nine years.

Cure Parkinson's

Cure Parkinson's is here for the cure – a cure for the fastest growing neurological condition in the world.

Parkinson's affects around ten million people worldwide. It is a progressive condition with over forty potential symptoms that can significantly impact a person's life, making the day-to-day activities that many take for granted a real challenge.

Current treatments only serve to provide temporary relief from symptoms and often bring troubling side effects. Cure Parkinson's refuses to accept this and is working with urgency to find new treatments with the potential to slow, stop or reverse the condition, offering those with Parkinson's the one thing they truly need: a cure.

They are discovering that drugs may already exist – treatments for other conditions – which could be adapted or repurposed as treatments for Parkinson's. As the drugs are already known to be safe, this could significantly reduce the time it takes to bring disease-modifying treatments to clinic for the Parkinson's community.

Cure Parkinson's has made significant progress towards their goal. But there's so much more to do. Curing Parkinson's needs world-class collaborative science involving researchers, clinicians, the pharmaceutical industry and, most importantly, people who are living with Parkinson's. This collaboration is at the heart of Cure Parkinson's' research programme.

Guy Deacon's journey through Africa has been an extraordinary undertaking. His work to raise awareness of Parkinson's worldwide has been relentless and inspiring, highlighting even further the urgent need for a cure. Cure Parkinson's is proud to have supported and be a benefactor of this project. this project. Together we will find a cure.

At the author's request your generous donations as a result of reading this book will be split between Cure Parkinson's and two further charities* who are working to support, inform and accelerate the search for cure for people affected by Parkinson's across the globe. Thank you.

Donate now:

*50% will be donated to Cure Parkinson's, registered Charity Number 1111816 (in England and Wales) and SCO44368 (in Scotland).

The Deacon Foundation

The Deacon Foundation was set up and registered as a charity in the UK to ensure that any proceeds from *Running on Empty* or the Channel 4 film of the same title are channelled to where it will make the biggest impact on people living with Parkinson's disease.

Throughout Africa, there are many individuals and small organisations who, with relatively modest incomes, are making a genuine difference to those who would otherwise have no help. They provide understanding and education and by so doing are de-stigmatising the condition. In some cases, they assist with the provision of medication, while others are lobbying health departments and hospitals. In all cases, they are improving the quality of life of those living with Parkinson's as well as their families and carers who are just as affected.

The Deacon Foundation is designed to maintain the momentum gained through the publication and sale of this book and the worldwide screening of the accompanying documentary. Grants will only ever be modest, but small amounts of money can go a very long way and in the case of the foundation, there are no overheads to speak of, so what is given is granted.

Running on Empty draws attention to Parkinson's in Africa, whereas the foundation, whilst initially focused on Africa, will support any low-level groups or individuals who are engaged in the battle against Parkinson's – wherever they may be.

The proceeds from the sale of this book will be shared between Cure Parkinson's, Parkinson's Africa and The Deacon Foundation. The three charities are not in competition with each other and are all very much in need of and greatly appreciate your support.

For more information visit: guydeacon.co.uk.

Registered Charity Number 1206038.
Kenley House, Chetnole, Sherborne, Dorset DT9 6NY

Parkinson's Africa

Parkinson's Africa exists to support and empower Africans impacted by Parkinson's disease (PD). This includes the family, friends, relatives and carers of those diagnosed.

We advocate on behalf of the Parkinson's community in Africa, fund, organise and support awareness campaigns, provide appropriate educational materials in local languages on Parkinson's disease in Africa and how to effectively manage the condition and offer support and activities. We help facilitate access to clinical services for people living with Parkinson's disease in Africa and we intend to continue looking for ways to help achieve an equitable medication pathway for Parkinson's patients in Africa. This, of course, would not be possible to achieve without our invaluable partners.

Parkinson's Africa is fully independent of any political or religious party. We do not directly provide medicine or in-depth clinical or medical services, but instead focus on raising awareness, educating, and supporting anyone in Africa affected by Parkinson's disease.

Parkinson's Africa was founded by Omotola Thomas, who was diagnosed with early-onset Parkinson's disease at the age of thirty-five in 2016.

For more information, visit: parkinsonsafrica.org